To Marg

I hope you find meaning in this book,

Please Don't Forget Me

Tom Pearson

Sincerely

Tom Pearson

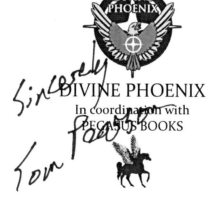

DIVINE PHOENIX
In coordination with
PEGASUS BOOKS

Pegasus Books
3338 San Marino Ave
San Jose, CA 95127
www.pegasusbooks.net

First Edition: April 2014

Published in North America by Divine Phoenix and Pegasus Books. For information, please contact Pegasus Books c/o Caprice De Luca, 3338 San Marino Ave, San Jose, CA 95127.

Library of Congress Cataloguing-In-Publication Data
Tom Pearson
Please Don't Forget Me/Tom Pearson– 1st ed
p. cm.
Library of Congress Control Number: 2014937674
ISBN – 978-0-9910993-8-2

1. HEALTH & FITNESS / Diseases / Alzheimer's & Dementia. 2. MEDICAL / Caregiving. 3. MEDICAL / Diseases / Brain. 4. SOCIAL SCIENCE / Death & Dying. 5. PSYCHOLOGY / Mental Health. 6. FAMILY & RELATIONSHIPS / Life Stages / Later Years. 7. FAMILY & RELATIONSHIPS / Love & Romance

10 9 8 7 6 5 4 3 2 1

Comments about *Please Don't Forget Me* and requests for additional copies, book club rates and author speaking appearances may be addressed to Tom Pearson at *tompleasedontforgetme@gmail.com* or Pegasus Books c/o Caprice De Luca, 3338 San Marino Ave, San Jose, CA, 95127, or you can send your comments and requests via e-mail to *laurasbooklist@aol.com*.

Also available as an eBook from Internet retailers and from Pegasus Books

Printed in the United States of America

Dedication

For the two loves of my life:

Lynne –
Thank you for the memories

Deborah –
Thank you for memories to come

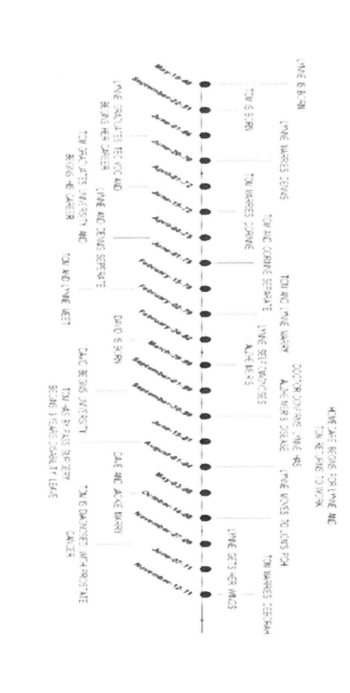

Please Don't Forget Me

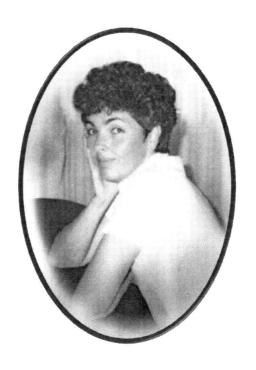

Table of Contents
Please Don't Forget Me
A Love Story

Prologue

It's fitting that I begin to write this story on the patio of our winter home in Indian Wells, with a glass of wine near at hand. Although my departed wife Lynne and I are from Winnipeg, Canada, Lynne enjoyed warm weather and wine much more than cold weather and Molson's Canadian beer.

And this is after all, Lynne's story. Tomorrow morning I will walk up the hill and visit her ashes, and we will talk for a while.

The impetus for this story comes from my dear friend Mary Sue who said, "You must share your story with others. It will give them hope." Mary Sue is a "fixer." She takes in rescue dogs and cares for them until they take over her house and a good part of her life. She also gives unselfishly to poor souls like me who end up on her doorstep now and then, in need of repair.

You will meet her later in this book. She is without a doubt my closest friend.

However, I am not certain that "hope" will be what you get from this book. This is not a happy story, although it has its "silver linings." It is a story of love and courage, of two people terribly, terribly in love and facing a common adversary.

But there is no happy ending. Alzheimer's disease kills people, pure and simple. There is no cure. It robs them of their memories, their minds and their dignity. I am not a religious person, and it is the ultimate irony that through caring for my dear wife, Lynne, as her disease progressed, I have come to believe unwaveringly in a "Higher Power."

That belief was brought into sharp focus recently when I read *The Alchemist* by Paulo Coelho. This is a lovely tale in which a young shepherd embarks upon his "Life Legend," his destiny. Throughout his journey the shepherd is tested in many ways, but as long as he "listens to his heart" the Universe conspires to help the shepherd achieve his legend.

The Universe is, of course, God. In the book and in our lives, God has many names: Allah, Jesus Christ, Buddha and on and on. The name isn't important.

The Alchemist caused me to reflect upon my own parallel experiences. My "Life Legend" was caring for Lynne until the end of her life. That was my destiny. The Universe helped me in some unexpected ways, and it took some time for me to understand that adversity sometimes had its benefits.

So I believe in this "Higher Power." But how Lynne's suffering factors into the Universe's plan remains an enigma to me. This fundamental question of faith has haunted humanity for as long as a belief in God has existed.

I know that I only have this one book in me. Though I hope that I have at least one more "Life Legend" to live. I need to "pay a few things forward" before I move on.

Tom Pearson
Indian Wells
November 2, 2012

Introduction

It is important that you understand where Lynne and I come from—our histories. Our life experiences and how we adapt to them truly define who we are. However, I have another reason for relating Lynne's history. It is just too easy to look at people who are at the end of their lives and all used up and forget the strong, vibrant people that they were.

Lynne was someone worth knowing. She was worth knowing before she got Alzheimer's disease, and she was worth knowing afterwards. Lynne should not be forgotten. So I intend to start this story at the beginning (that would be at birth!) for both Lynne and me, and for that innocent bystander in this saga, our son David.

Lynne's history is incomplete. I know a lot about Lynne, but I can't possibly know everything. And there are likely things that she just wanted to keep to herself. You will see her through my eyes.

But remember that Lynne's fingerprints are all over me. I have known Lynne for thirty-four years—over half my lifetime. During our years together she shaped me just as surely as an artisan shapes clay. I think that my perception of Lynne is very close to how she saw herself. The main difference would be that I loved her far more than she loved herself. I still do.

I've tried to relate my own history as honestly as possible. There were times when I wasn't a particularly good person. Yet I grew and changed, in a large measure thanks to Lynne. Lynne made me a better person than I ever expected to be.

So you will see Lynne's history until we met, my history until we met and our lives together before and after Lynne was diagnosed with Alzheimer's disease. The facts relating to Lynne and me on a personal level are exactly that. They comprise a true story.

Everything else is based on the world and its people as seen through my eyes. What you will read is reality seen through my eyes. My perceptions are exactly that. They are not statements of fact and I earnestly hope that the people who pop up in this book are not distressed by how I see them. Except for Lynne's mother. And she left us years ago.

Lynne, before Tom

The Lynne I knew could have been a storybook heroine. She was beautiful, she was funny, and she was oh, so smart! And as you will learn later, Lynne had the heart of a lion. She was very, very brave.

This is Lynne's story before she met me, as best as I can piece it together.

Lynne was born on May 10, 1948 and her name was Marjorie Lynne Foster. Her father and mother were Jack and Marjorie Foster, and she had one brother, five years older, also named Jack (full name Jack Carson Foster).

There was not a lot of originality in the Foster family when it came to naming children; the first son was named after his father, and the first daughter was named after her mother. I suppose additional children beyond Jack and Lynne would have required some moments of inspiration, but that never happened.

Although her brother went by "Jack," the same as his father, Lynne did not use her mother's name. She did not use it when I met her, and I know that she hadn't used it for more than a decade before we met. That fact speaks volumes about the relationship between the two women. Lynne's mother was a difficult and sometimes cruel woman. More about that later.

Lynne spent the first two years of her life in an area of Winnipeg known as Riverview, not far from where I live now. Even in 1948 it was a well-established area with large trees, quiet shady streets and large homes, some dating back to the early 1900's.

The main difference between Riverview then and now (other than some modern architecturally designed in-fill homes like mine that long-time residents describe euphemistically as "controversial") is that Riverview lacked flood protection. As the name implies, the community sits next to a river. More specifically, it sits next to the Red

River, which drains the vast plains to the south of Winnipeg.

In 1950, after the one-two-three punch of heavy snowfall, a rapid snowmelt and rain, the sleepy old Red River turned into a monster that left downtown Winnipeg under water, and flooded the Foster family's home to roof level.

The elder Fosters decided that they did not want to experience the Red River's wrath again anytime soon, so they moved to a then-new subdivision known as River Heights. Their new home was nowhere near a river, but as the name implied, it was on higher ground.

The Red River floodwaters had not reached this area in 1950 and I am certain that this gave considerable impetus to the sale of the tract homes that sprang up in the area after the flood. At the time, the area had all the charm (not!) of most new subdivisions with spindly trees and little or no shade, but it has since matured into a very desirable area, despite poor soil conditions and the resulting foundation problems in some of the homes.

So this modest bungalow in River Heights is where Lynne grew up.

Early photographs of Lynne show a beautiful baby with dark hair, huge brown eyes and an enigmatic little smile, almost as though she were saying, "Hmm, this is nice!" All of these characteristics followed her into adulthood. Much later, when Lynne was in the more severe phases of Alzheimer's disease the smile resurfaced. I called it her "Mona Lisa" smile, and I took comfort when I saw it, because I knew that she felt happy and safe.

As Lynne grew, photographs show a little girl that can best be described as "cute as a bug." The smile broadened and dimples appeared. The dark hair was worn in curls around those big brown eyes of hers, which now had a mischievous twinkle (I always loved Lynne's eyes. I swear that when I looked into them, I could see clear into her beautiful soul).

I think from looking at early photos that Lynne adored her older brother Jack when they were young, although the five year age difference may have pushed them apart a little bit during their teens. Or it may be that their mother was conspiring to divide them even then. Lynne's mother was a very needy person, and she was not above telling either Lynne or her brother Jack lies about one another so that only she was the object of their affection.

I do know that Lynne's mother's ploy didn't work, at least in the long-term. Lynne loved her brother and took pride in his accomplishments throughout her lifetime. That doesn't mean that everything was perfect! Jack did things that annoyed the crap out of Lynne now and then and I am certain that Lynne annoyed Jack equally from time to time.

Such are the dynamics of families. But the most important dynamic was a life-long affection for one another.

Lynne's mother had another less-than-desirable trait that likely shaped both siblings, and that was her dissatisfaction with her socio-economic status. Lynne's mother to my knowledge never worked outside the home (not uncommon during those times) and her husband Jack was the sole bread winner.

They lived in a neighbourhood where many families were considerably more affluent and had larger homes. Lynne always used to tell me fairly scornfully that, "we never had any money when we grew up."

I think that she was unconsciously parroting something that her mother had told her, something that demeaned her father, who was actually a very good provider and steward of his modest lower-middle management salary. I know this because Jack senior was able to retire comfortably at a relatively early age and continue to maintain his membership at Elmhurst (a prestigious golf club) while purchasing a new car every five years.

Lynne's father when I knew him was a delightful man (although a bit of a bigot) who coped with his wife by golfing extensively in the summer months, and walking to Salisbury House each day for a protracted breakfast. All of the waitresses there fussed over him when he was alone, and gave him a wide berth when his wife inflicted her presence on them and her husband.

I know that Lynne loved her father dearly, and did not love her mother. She tried, but she couldn't do it. But her mother's dissatisfaction with their economic status did instill in her children a need to succeed on a financial level, which they did. Jack and Lynne were both very intelligent and driven people.

Lynne started grade school in September of 1954 and graduated from high school in June of 1965. She apparently did very well in her early school years, even skipping a grade before she lapsed into that sort of ennui that sometimes plagues students in their teen years. In any event, Lynne graduated high school with middling marks, well below her potential.

I often wonder whether her mother's constant berating and her demeaning attitude didn't somehow rob Lynne of the enthusiasm that she needed to succeed at that time of her life. After graduating from high school, Lynne enrolled in Tec Voc (a vocational school) in September of 1966 where she took a one year program in accounting and clerical skills.

This was apparently all her mother felt that she was capable of, notwithstanding that by this time her brother Jack had attained a Commerce degree from the University of Manitoba.

I honestly believe that Lynne's mother had simply decided that she would not allow Lynne to surpass her own modest achievements in life, out of a combination of vindictiveness and a prejudice against women in the workplace. This was a shame. Lynne was one of the smartest people that I have ever met; much smarter than me, and I have two degrees in engineering.

Lynne could grasp concepts instantly, and get to the core of an issue with the speed and accuracy of a heat-seeking missile. Years later, when I called her ex-husband Dennis (you will meet him later) to let him know that Lynne had Alzheimer's disease, his first sadly uttered words were, "But she was so smart! How can this be?" His second words were, "Is her mother dead yet?" He detested Lynne's mother as much as I did. Two husbands can't be all wrong.

Lynne graduated from Tec Voc a year later in June of 1966, and began a career at Great West Life the same year. I was not surprised to find a copy of her first pay stub in her papers (her first cheque was for $115.00 per month and after deductions she netted $99.87). Lynne was a very organized person. In fact, she kept me organized for most of our married life.

Once Lynne moved away from home, she did very well in the work world, which was a far more positive environment for her. Lynne rose to the position of executive secretary to the personnel director before she left Great West Life in 1975.

During that time she met Irene Hay and the two became life-long friends. Irene was there for Lynne through the thick and the thin. As I write this, I realize that I need to connect with Irene again and make certain that she is doing well. Such is the debt of that kind of friendship—you need to be there and provide help when you are needed.

Lynne then became a co-proprietor in an antique shop called Sauterelle Imports in a trendy area of Winnipeg known as Osborne Village. She was only in business for a year, but she made many good friends while she was there. Lynne then became involved in commercial real estate from 1976, until 1978.

During the time that Lynne was at Great West Life, she met her first husband Dennis, and they were married in June, 1970. At the time, Dennis worked for the railway. After

Lynne and he were married he began dabbling in real estate and at one point had over 20 rental properties. He eventually became a broker, went into real estate full time and was quite successful.

Dennis separated from Lynne in 1977. Lynne never talked much about the separation, but after talking to Dennis once, I believe I got a glimmer of what happened. Lynne's mother had a firm hold on Lynne at the time, and she never liked Dennis. She called Lynne on a daily basis, doing her best to sow seeds of dissent and upsetting Lynne. She basically made their married life a living hell and almost caused Lynne to have a breakdown. Eventually Dennis had enough, and he walked.

And then Lynne met me.

Tom, before Lynne

I was born on September 22, 1951 and my name is Thomas Robert Pearson, but everyone calls me Tom. My parents' names were Robert and Margaret Pearson. I have one sister, Lynn Margaret who is one year older than me.

Apparently the naming convention in the Pearson household was only slightly more original than that of the Foster family. I was named after my grandfather (Thomas) and my father (Robert). My folks did go a little wild with my sister, whose first name was an original selection, and whose second name is after our mother Margaret.

I spent the first thirteen years of my life in St. Norbert, which at the time was almost rural in nature and barely part of Winnipeg. The 1950 flood also affected the Pearson family—I just wasn't there yet. At the time of the flood my mother and father owned and operated some tourist cabins just south of where our family home was subsequently built. The cabins were flooded to above the roof line. Some of them just floated away.

Afterwards my father and mother sold the cabins. Dad went to work for the provincial government (that's like the state government, for you Americans) and Mom became a book-keeper for a tile contractor. They built a new home just up the road from the cabins, on a little higher ground. But not high enough that we didn't need a canoe to get to the house during another flood in 1960.

I started grade school just before my sixth birthday in September, 1957. Believe it or not, I attended a one-room school house for grades one through seven until the end of grade four. Our teacher was a lovely young creature and I am certain that every boy in the room was in love with her. We all listened raptly and did whatever she asked, without question. For some reason I cannot recall her name. It may have been Miss Obudynski.

After the 1960 flood the provincial government finally got serious about flood protection and construction of the Winnipeg floodway began. The floodway diverts floodwaters from the south around Winnipeg and has saved the city countless times since it was built. I'll tell you a little story about a flood later in the book.

Our little one-room school was right in the path of the floodway, so it was demolished and all of us kids had to attend a much larger school in St. Norbert, where the student population was predominantly French speaking.

This assimilation did not go smoothly, at least initially. I knew enough French (my grandma was French) to know when the French kids were insulting me in their language and a few fights ensued. At that time I was a bit of a porker, but I was large for my age and I had some experience brawling with my older sister who tormented me incessantly (she was pretty tough for a girl).

That resulted in some detentions, of course. Our home-room teacher was another pretty lady named Miss Lord, and she treated me so well that I didn't mind. Grades six and seven were another story. In grade six we had a nun named Sister Sabourin who terrorized us with a wooden pointer and in grade seven we had a Mister Bosc, who had a short fuse and liked to use the strap.

Anyway, after a little while we kids from the one-room school house adapted to our new environment. Friendships were forged, we were accepted and all was well.

My childhood was wonderful during that time. Both of my parents worked and as a result they could afford to build a lakefront cottage in Ontario. My mother would take most of the summer off and spend it with us kids at the lake, so summer was full of fishing, swimming and water-skiing, and exploring the lake in a canoe with a close buddy that lived next door.

I only have two negative memories of that time. My dad liked to garden and he would plant a huge vegetable garden on our property. I had to weed it and to this day I detest gardening.

The other memory has most folks in stitches when I tell it, but it was pretty scary for us kids at the time. Our folks went out on New Year's Eve and left us kids alone. Just around mid-night a drunk came knocking on our door, and he wouldn't leave. We could see him through the glass in the door.

We lived in an isolated area and we were very frightened. So I went and got my single-shot shotgun and popped a shell into the chamber. The drunk saw this through the door, sobered up immediately and high-tailed it! It turned out he was a friend of my dad's, but we didn't know that at the time. My dad thought it was pretty funny. I disagreed.

Things changed big-time after grade seven. My dad quit his job with the government and he and a partner bought a trucking company and we moved to a rural community called Sturgis, Saskatchewan. Which is in the middle of nowhere.

Actually, things were amazing in Sturgis! For recreation we used to shoot rats at the grain elevators near the house. At night a buddy and I would sneak out and hot wire one of my parent's cars and go to one of the many Ukrainian socials in the area, where we would drink moonshine and flirt with girls—underage driving, underage drinking and girls. What more could a teenage boy want?

Unfortunately, my dad's trucking company went bankrupt, we moved back to St. Norbert and Mom went back to work. After a while the cabin in Ontario was sold and my parents bought a hardware store in a small town called Morris, Manitoba.

My social life was great, but money was tight and things were not good between my parents. After school, I worked in the hardware store (for free) as well as holding down a job pumping gas and repairing truck tires for spending money.

I managed to save enough money to buy a pretty hot car (a 58 Impala hardtop v-8 with three carbs) which I promptly totalled by flipping it end-over-end. Amazingly, no one was hurt. I sold the wreck and bought an old Buick. Not my first choice, but it was cheap. And as it turned out, my mother needed a car.

About that time, my father decided that he needed to go to British Columbia (B.C.) to "find his fortune," or maybe he just wanted to leave Mom. Anyway, he left Mom to tend to the store, and I worked hard to help her.

I don't remember my sister doing much, but I do remember her cooking some meals. To be fair, my sister had to work a lot harder than I did to get through school. I just kind of sailed through with minimal effort, easily achieving good grades.

When a mechanic "friend" of my father's came out to fix the Buick, my mother had an affair with him. I don't think she knew that I knew, but kids aren't stupid.

I guess she had just had enough with my father leaving. I didn't like it, but I didn't hate her for it either. I loved my Mom and by this time I didn't like my dad much. I have never said a word to anyone about this until now.

By then, I had a steady girlfriend named Corinne, and I thought that I was in love. So when my mother announced that they were selling the store and that we were moving to Vancouver Island, B. C. to reunite with my father, I did not want to go.

I was sixteen at the time and had just completed grade eleven. My objections were met with minimal resistance. I obtained permission from the provincial school officials to challenge the grade twelve supplementary exams at the end of summer. I boarded with a family in Morris who had a spare room in their basement and I holed up there and read all of the grade twelve textbooks.

I wanted to go into mechanical engineering, so I had to complete all of the physics and chemistry labs to satisfy the admission requirements. To this day I am eternally grateful to my science teacher Mr. Coates, who let me into the school to do the labs, waited patiently for me to complete them, and then marked them. He was a good teacher and he is a good man.

Anyway, after six weeks of intensive study I wrote the exams and met the entrance requirements (barely) for engineering. I was still sixteen when I entered the university.

My folks covered my room and board for the first year—only fair in my mind, as my mother had taken my car to B.C.!—and I took out a student loan for tuition and books. After that, I was pretty much on my own. I bought an old Chevy on the verge of extinction and got a part time job (graveyard shift) pumping gas for spending money. The graveyard shift meshed well with university. I could study between customers and turn off the pumps and catch a little sleep in the early morning hours.

I never felt hard done by. I had enough money to live, run a car and for a social life. And I was always able to make good money during the summer. The only time I got a little rankled is when I heard that my parents had set my sister up with a beauty parlor in B.C., when they had given me very little help. Daddy's girl.

After such a condensed version of grade twelve, I studied hard during the first year of engineering and did well. By the second year I needed to let off some steam. I rented a house with three buddies, and it was party central.

My marks plummeted and I got a D in algebra and an F in calculus. That brought focus to my studies and by graduation I had brought my marks up to the level where I could get into grad school if I wanted to. As it turned out, I did want to (much later).

The really great part of my year at "party central" was that I forged lifelong friendships, and ironically all of us "party animals" turned out pretty well.

During this time I would go back to Morris to visit Corinne on weekends until she completed high school and then we dated while she was in Winnipeg completing her nursing training. We broke up a couple of times, but reconciled, and we were married after I graduated from Mechanical Engineering in 1972. We were both twenty at the time. In hindsight, this was much too young.

Nurses were in high demand when Corinne graduated, but the economy was slow and it took me a while to find work. After a couple of failed attempts and a lot of persistence I landed at a consulting engineering firm doing work that I enjoyed, and I was successful.

Corinne and I bought our first house (a small bi-level backing onto a river) and I did some renovations that added a fair bit of value. We sold the house and upgraded to a larger one in a very nice area of the city called Southdale.

I worked hard and travelled a fair amount. Things should have been great between us, but they were not. Corinne never said anything about it and to be honest I think I just ignored the lack of depth in our relationship. I loved my work and I spent a lot of time doing it.

Things went askew when I caught Corinne with her boyfriend (I learned afterward that she had been seeing him even before we bought the new house). We tried counselling, but I was very angry and I don't think Corinne was interested in reconciling.

She left for work one day and didn't come home. A few days later I came home from work to an empty house. All of our furniture (except for a dining room suite and a bed) was gone. It was June of 1976.

Despite the circumstances, Corinne wanted her share and then some. She already had all the furniture and had drained the bank account, but she wanted half the house, half my pension, a cabin lot that I had acquired (I think that her brother had his eye on that) and one of the cars.

After some fairly acrimonious negotiations which enriched a couple of lawyers she kept her pension and I kept mine, we split the house and I gave up an Audi in exchange for the cabin lot. That was a good deal. That car was nothing but trouble. I have not seen Corinne since and I don't want to, ever.

After that I was a young, bitter man with a great job, good money and no conscience. I had many relationships with women, some of which ended in tears. I would usually have a "steady" girlfriend, but if anyone else attractive came along, that was OK too.

I once ran into an ex-neighbour who lived across the street from Corinne and me when we split up. She was in a bar, along with her very attractive younger sister. She said, "I felt so bad when your wife came in the middle of the day and took all the furniture!" Several drinks later the sister was so sympathetic that she took me home to bed with her. I had no shame.

I filled in what little spare time I had building a fairly nice cabin at the lake in Ontario and fishing. Sometimes I would take a girl out there with me. I suppose in hindsight that I was trying to even the score with women in general. I am not proud of the man I was back then...

And then I met Lynne.

Sparks Fly

I suppose that I owe meeting Lynne to a co-worker named Jim Aitkens. But these days I prefer to think that the Universe despite my terrible behaviour, had decided to give me another chance.

Jim was also "between wives." He wandered into my office one Friday afternoon and said, "Why don't you come to the Winnipeg Ski Club with me tonight? There's a dance and there will be a party afterward." I said, "Jim, I don't ski." To which he responded, "That's not why we're going." Aha.

Jim was a colourful character. He was an over-the-hill party animal that had his own plane. He had a bad back and sometimes spent his afternoons lying on the floor of his office with his head propped up on some books, dictating letters. Anyway, I went along...

When I walked into the Ski Club, Lynne was sitting at a table selling tickets (she confided in me a long time afterwards that she was selling tickets so she could check out the men as they came in the door). Our eyes met and it was as though a shock ran through me! Her smile lit up the room.

Looking back at that moment, I honestly believe that it was love at first sight. Even in the jaded, womanizing state that I was in at that time, I knew a beautiful, intelligent woman when I saw her. We spent the evening dancing and talking, went to the after-party and then went home together. I was enchanted. I was drawn to her by her beauty, but her keen intellect and vivaciousness captivated me.

We continued to see one-another and it wasn't too long before I decided it was time to say good-bye to the other two girls I was seeing at the time. One break-up was pretty clean, other than dodging a fair-sized vase that crashed into the wall next to my head.

The other was kind of creepy, almost stalker-like. She would call me in the middle of the night and make lewd suggestions over the phone. A new unlisted telephone number fixed that one. I didn't want any of those calls while Lynne was in the room!

Interestingly, Lynne and I had kind of a "don't ask, don't tell" attitude about our previous marriages and other relationships. I had fallen in love with her and I just didn't want to know. And thankfully, neither did Lynne.

A while after we met, Lynne went off to Mexico with a girlfriend on a pre-arranged vacation. I missed her terribly, and when she came back I asked her to move in with me, and to consider marriage if things went well. We had both been through failed marriages and some caution was in order.

Thus began an idyllic year. At the time, I lived on the top floor of an apartment building in an area called "The Gates" near downtown. Lynne put her furniture in storage and moved there. In the summer, we went to a new restaurant once or twice a week. We often walked.

We went to the cabin on weekends, where we would troll around the bay in the morning until we caught breakfast. Then we worked on the cabin all day and barbequed dinner.

In the winter we would cross-country ski and then go for brunch. It was all very romantic. But for me more than anything else, it was the exhilaration of having conversations with this fascinating, intelligent creature that I had fallen hopelessly in love with. I loved Lynne's mind, her intellect and her smile.

During the summer that Lynne moved in with me, her brother Jack came to visit us. He was going through town on business and he wanted to check me out. At the time, Jack was a senior executive in the food industry and he was a no-nonsense guy, used to having his way. I was managing multi-million dollar construction contracts, so I wasn't used to taking crap from anyone either.

So we danced around a little and then he decided I was OK and I decided he was OK. Then I discovered the purpose of his visit and at the same time came face-to-face with just ow poisonous Jack and Lynne's mother was. He told me what she had said.

"Tom will never marry Lynne. He'll just use her and be on his way." He looked at me closely and said, "I don't think that's going to happen." He was protecting his little sister.

The first thought that ran through my mind after the shock subsided was *How could a mother wish that on her child?* The second, less charitable thought was *What an evil bitch!* Thus began an era of collaboration between Lynne and Jack about the lies that their mother told them to turn them against one another (and me).

Lynne and I were married in the United Church on Broadway across from the parliament buildings on February 2, 1979. It was a typical cold sunny Winnipeg day and the sun streamed through the church's stained glass windows and lit up Lynne's face.

It was a small wedding, just a few close friends and Lynne's brother Jack and his wife. Afterwards we went to Victor's Restaurant in the Village for dinner, where we had reserved a room. Lynne and I had already been to Barbados at Christmas for kind of an advance honeymoon. After the wedding we went to the Florida Gulf Coast, just for good measure.

I loved Lynne from the moment I first laid eyes upon her. We married for life. If my first wife hadn't left me, I never would have met Lynne. Sometimes things happen for a reason.

And we lived happily ever after. But remember, "Happily Ever After" takes a lot of work.

Our family: Ups and downs, and ups

After we married, Lynne quit real estate and became the chief operating officer (COO) of the Pearson household. We wanted to start a family. Lynne was thirty years old when we married, and I was twenty-seven, so we needed to get busy.

As an aside: *Lynne always worried a bit about the fact that she was a little more than three years older than me. She was concerned that she would begin to look "old" before I did. It didn't concern me in the least. Lynne was pretty, but that wasn't the reason that I loved her. Anyway, she aged well and she always looked much better than I did. I guess, other than Alzheimer's, she had good genes.*

We figured that if we were going to have a family, we'd better have a house. My debacle with Corinne had set me back a bit, and so had Lynne's divorce. I honestly believe that old adage that the only winners in a divorce are the lawyers!

So we decided that some "sweat equity" was in order. We bought property on a street called Old River Road in a rural area north of Winnipeg and we began to build a house.

Lynne's first challenge as COO was materials procurement and participation in construction of our new home. Lynne was a force to be reckoned with! She bought and delivered lumber. She brought lunches and dinners to the site, she installed insulation and vapour barrier and primed windows and doors. Not too shabby for a tall, slender woman who looked more like a fashion model than a construction worker!

Often I was at work while all this was happening. Although I used my vacation to start construction of the house, the construction time far exceeded my available vacation time, so I worked on the house during evenings and weekends. I once arrived home to find Lynne toe-to-toe with our finish-painting contractor. She was telling him, "If you do a half-assed job, I'll write you a half-assed cheque!"

And that's what he ended up settling for. When Lynne said something, she meant it.

Lynne was also a keen negotiator. I used to say jokingly that she could make a dollar scream. When Lynne was assembling the appliance order for the house she cruised various stores looking for demo products and unobtrusive scratch and dent pieces. She finally found what she believed to be the optimum combination at a mid-size store on Henderson Highway.

She had the store manager follow her around pricing the items after making it abundantly clear that price was paramount. Then Lynne looked him in the eye and said, "This is your first and only chance to make a deal. How much will you give me off these prices if I take everything now? Cash." Another fifteen percent came of the top, and Lynne had her dream kitchen, below budget.

Something else happened over that period. Lynne's dad got wind of what we were doing, and he began to come over to help her. Lynne was estranged from her mother at the time (for very good reasons) and she was worried that this would allow her mother to penetrate her life again.

But Lynne loved her dad and could not turn him away. The two of them spent many happy hours working together. Lynne's mother seldom cooked, so her dad was in his glory scarfing down the home-cooked meals that Lynne brought to the job-site. Lynne was an excellent cook.

Lynne's brother, Jack, and his family came to visit and stayed about a week just after the house was completed. Lynne prepared several feasts for them, and then we went to the cabin to swim, water ski and party. Jack's kids were in their early teens, and they had a blast. It reminded me of my time at my parent's cabin when I was young.

When the house was done, we had a stunning, large Tudor style bungalow with a family room with a fireplace, a double attached garage, a sun deck and a screened patio— the kind of house that would only fit on a large rural lot. A lovely home.

Unfortunately, as Lynne put it, "we decided that we were city mice, not country mice." It was a long commute to work for me, and Lynne felt isolated out there alone. If you forgot a quart of milk, it was a forty minute trip to get one. So we resolved to move back to the city. Another lesson learned...

Using her real estate experience, Lynne marketed our rural home. She used to get me to show the home. She said, "You could sell ice to Eskimos. People just instinctively trust you." I took that as a great compliment from Lynne. It meant that she had total trust in me as well.

We sold the home to a young couple that was just starting out, a little like us. They showed up in an old beat up car and it was obvious that they didn't have enough money to buy the house. I treated them with respect and gave them a tour of our home anyway.

It turned out that while they didn't have the money, the young fellow's Ukrainian Baba did. Cash, no mortgage required! We did a little better than a break-even on the house, and I was happy to see it go to people who would fill it with family and joy.

Of course, during that time we had to find another home to move to. Lynne (ever the entrepreneur) decided that our best option was to find a "fixer-upper" in a good location. She still had some close friends in the real estate business and she had those friends scouting properties for us.

Lynne called me at work one day and said, "Jack Cooper has found a place for us. The sign's not up yet and he says it looks terrible, but it is way under value. Can you meet me there?" I hustled over to the house to meet the realtor and Lynne and in we went. What happened next caused both of us great sadness.

The owners of the house had separated, however, they hadn't told their teenage son that they were calling it quits and selling the house. The son had skipped school and came crawling out of bed as we arrived, wondering what was up.

Before we could explain, one of those rare coincidences occurred. The sign company arrived and was erecting a "For Sale" on the front lawn as the son stared out the living room window. He put two and two together and began to sob.

Lynne consoled him as best she could, but she was spitting mad when we left. Even with all the things that her mother had done to her, she could not understand how parents could do that to their child.

But we bought the house

The house was not nearly as bad as it looked. It was much larger than we needed though—a large bungalow with four bedrooms and two baths on the main floor and finished basement with a rec-room, another bedroom and a laundry room.

It needed new paint inside and out, some exterior detailing, new floor coverings throughout, new appliances and countertops, an upgrade of the two existing bathrooms and a new bathroom in the basement. A piece of cake, right? A pattern had been established and Lynne and I began to knock off the to-do list according to our areas of expertise.

But there were time constraints! Lynne and I, despite our best efforts had been unable to conceive a child. So we decided that we would adopt, and placed our names on the waiting list. It was a very long list, about four years back then. I imagine it is much longer now.

Back then as now, there was significant prejudice against aboriginal people. Our social worker told us that if we were prepared to accept an infant with some aboriginal heritage in his/her history the wait would be much shorter. This was a no brainer for both of us, notwithstanding that we knew that both sets of grandparents had a strong bias against aboriginals.

The irony of this was not lost on me. My dear grandmother, my father's mother, who in a large part raised me while my mother worked, was French Canadian, but he had to be at least one-eighth aboriginal based on our family tree and her appearance. Anyway, we agreed to change our criteria and our names rocketed to the top of the list. Not long after, we got a call that changed our lives.

Our son David was born on February 24, 1982 and he came home with us on March 9, 1982. He was just five and a half pounds at the time, an alert little thing who stared at us inquisitively with brown eyes and then seemed to think, *Hmm, I think that they'll do* and gave us a smile! It's hard to believe that he has grown to be the fine young man he is today. Like me, he has Lynne's fingerprints all over him.

I know that we were by no means unique in this regard, but bringing a new-borne baby home when you have had no experience with them is a challenge. They don't come with instruction books, and they can't talk so you don't know what they want.

They are happy, crying or sleeping. We learned quickly that happy and sleeping were good, and crying usually (but not always) meant "feed me" or "change my diaper." But Dave quickly got to know us and we got to know him and things went well.

I used to feed and change him in the middle of the night early on before he began to sleep through morning. One of my fondest memories was feeding him in the rocking chair while staring out the window on a typically still Winnipeg winter night, watching the huge snowflakes fall slowly to the ground. It was very peaceful.

Life was good in our new home. Lynne stayed home to raise David. We had a trip to Maui when David was about one year old. We had lots of parties with friends and family.

A year after David was born I changed jobs. Consulting engineering involved a fair amount of travel, and there was always pressure to move to some godforsaken place in Africa to manage a project. You could only say no so many times. So I got a senior engineering job with the City of Winnipeg, and I ended up staying there for 28 years.

One of the drawbacks of this change was an end to the three day weekends that I was able to take over the summer. The long drive to our cabin in Ontario made two day stays untenable. So when Dave was about three we sold our cabin and a great debate arose in our family about how to spend the money.

Our Chief Financial Officer (that was Lynne) wanted to pay off the house and invest the balance. I won that argument! We went to Maui for a month, we bought a new car and we paid down the mortgage. We made friends while we were in Maui and celebrated Dave's third birthday with them while we were with there. Good memories.

There weren't many kids Dave's age in our neighbourhood and by the time he was five he was hanging out with fifteen and sixteen year olds in the neighbour's driveway. They had sort of adopted him as their mascot.

So we had a new home built in an area called Island Lakes, and we moved one more time. Our new home was Lynne's "dream house." Despite the fact that it only had three bedrooms, it was much larger than our old home, with vaulted ceilings in the living and dining rooms, a separate family room with a fireplace, and a huge kitchen with a separate hexagonal eating nook with glass on three sides.

I added a sunroom for Lynne and finished part of the basement for Dave. The bonus for me was a spacious double attached garage, which I promptly insulated and heated (can you say *man-cave*?).

Our house in Island Lakes was to be our home for twenty-one years. The bookends on our life there were to be Dave leaving for kindergarten the first fall after we moved and the cake cutting ceremony after Dave and Jackie's wedding.

In between we had many good times. Max and Shirley moved in next door and Lynne and Shirley were the best of friends. But there were storm clouds on the horizon—on two fronts.

When David was born, Lynne decided that it wasn't right not to let her mother back into her life. Lynne felt that her mother should be able to see her grandchild, even though there was a risk that Lynne's mother's poison would creep back into our lives.

I always took the attitude that these types of decisions were Lynne's, not mine. But I had grave concerns because from where I sat, Lynne's mother was a monster. Sadly, I wasn't mistaken. Before too long, Lynne was getting two to three calls a day from her mother, each an hour or so long and filled with lies about Lynne's brother and his family, disparaging remarks about me and long discussions on what poor parents we were.

Lynne was a strong woman, but she could never stand up to her mother. I guess a childhood of emotional abuse made it just too hard for her to do it. So Lynne asked me to call a family meeting and put some boundaries on the relationship, which I did.

I explained that Lynne needed her mom to cut down on the call times and to stop disparaging people we loved when she called. She looked at me and said, "I didn't think you had it in you." I held my tongue. Then she looked at Lynne and said, "Are you going to let him run your life?" To Lynne's credit, she looked her mother in the eye and said, "This is my choice. I asked Tom to talk to you."

I was so proud of Lynne at that moment. The Devil had called her out, and Lynne hadn't blinked.

Lynne's father had a very sad look on his face, and I knew why. After that, we never saw Lynne's mother again. She severed all relationships and consequently we seldom saw Lynne's father either. Those meetings were few and in secret. Lynne's mother did not tell Lynne when her father died. We heard about it after the fact from her brother Jack. Lynne did not attend her mother's funeral when she passed. Sadly, we were both relieved to see her gone.

The other storm cloud had to do with Lynne and my relationship. At one point Lynne became dissatisfied with life in general and depressed, and she decided that it was because of me. We talked about what was wrong. We argued. We analyzed.

But it all came back to me. After a while, it dawned on me that this wasn't just my problem and that maybe Lynne was suffering from clinical depression. She was very hard to live with and you couldn't win an argument with her. Lynne was just too damned smart.

It must have been very hard for our son David to hear all this going on and wondering what was going to happen to our family. Once I just walked away from an argument, and Lynne got so angry that she threw the remote control for the TV at the back of my head. It made a dent in the wall, which I never repaired. It was still there when I sold the house.

Finally I said that I had had enough and I moved into the guest room. I told her that we needed to get help or our marriage was over. Lynne was a proud, determined woman. It took her six months, but eventually she relented and we went for counselling. The doctor diagnosed her depression and treated it, and all was well. We were back in love. And I thanked God.

Things got back to normal, and normal was pretty good. By that time I had completed a Master's Degree in environmental engineering and advanced to a senior management role, responsible for the city's water supply system, land drainage and a few other things. I also served on the boards of a couple of industry organizations.

I worked hard, but I had seven weeks of vacation a year and Winnipeg is cold in the winter! Lynne and I would go to the gulf coast of Florida in November, take a winter vacation somewhere nice in January and then attend a winter board meeting in February. If the board meeting was in a nice spot we would tack on an extra week of vacation. We were very fortunate. And we were very happy.

In 1997 Winnipeg had had another of its epic floods. They called this one the "flood of the century." But it is what happened before the flood that caused me terrible grief and anguish.

We had a late winter storm followed by warm weather. It was as though someone had thrown a switch. The snow began to melt at a record pace, and large ponds of water quickly accumulated in the remaining ditches in Winnipeg. Such a ditch exists in front of an elementary school in north Winnipeg, and the kids were drawn to it like a magnet. What none of us knew was that a terrible hazard lurked at the bottom of this ditch.

You see, in order to drain the ditch an eighteen inch diameter culvert had been installed at a steep angle down from the bottom of the ditch to a large land drainage sewer below. Even though the water above the culvert was at least two feet deep, it created a large whirlpool that made the children curious.

A young boy named Adam, about fourteen years old got too close and was drawn into the vortex and down into the labyrinth of pipes below our city streets. It was April 22, 1997. It took us several days to find his body, several miles away on one of the trash racks installed in the sewer system to keep large debris out of the pipes. The crew that found the boy was traumatized.

Shortly after Adam's family was notified that we had found his body, I received a call from City Hall. Adam's father wanted to talk to someone. He needed to understand what had happened to his son. Would I do it? I agreed, but for the first time in my life I felt I might not be up to the task before me. I kept thinking of my own son, and what had happened to Adam.

Adam's father arrived and I escorted him to my office and closed the door. He was very quiet; reserved. I had arranged for staff to prepare some drawings and a sketch to illustrate the situation and I began to explain it to Adam's father. He began sobbing uncontrollably. You see, the pipe

was only eighteen inches in diameter, and Adam was a big
boy.

I wrapped my arms around Adam's father and held him
for several moments, until he settled down—two grown
men, clinging to one another, in a city office. When I
finished my explanation he asked me, "Did he suffer?"

I couldn't lie to him. I said that I did not know, but in
all likelihood the trauma of passing through the culvert (it
was about ten feet long) had caused him to lose
consciousness and he would have drowned shortly after
that. I asked him if I could have someone drive him home,
and he said thank you, but no. When he left me he was
walking as though in a trance.

I was numb for the rest of the day. I cancelled all of my
meetings. I could barely function as the scene with Adam's
father played over and over in my mind. Finally, I left work
early and went home to Lynne. I told her my story over a
single malt scotch straight-up, and then wept quietly in her
arms.

After that, there was no time to dwell on young Adam.
The flood was coming and we needed to get ready.

There is a big difference between fighting a flood and
say, fighting a fire. With a fire, there is an adrenalin rush
and then it's over. With a flood (at least on the plains),
there is intense planning and preparation before the water
arrives, followed by several weeks of reacting to unforeseen
circumstances (weather, dyke breaches and the like) and
then clean-up.

All the while, you have to feed the two information
gluttons—the media and the politicians. The adrenalin rush
quickly turns into an epic marathon. In Winnipeg we've
done it so many times that we've got it down pretty well.
We actually have a flood manual and a cadre of external
resources we tap into to help us through the bad ones.

And believe me, 1997 was one of the bad ones—the
worst flood we had faced in one hundred years. I was one of
an army of people at work to save Winnipeg from the rising

waters. We all worked gruelling hours—twelve hour days, seven days a week for weeks on end as we watched Grand Forks to the south of us go under water.

I had some significant responsibilities so I would often end up at City Hall for meetings. More than once I forgot where I had parked my car, only to discover, when I finally found it that I had locked my keys in it. I would call Lynne and she would meet me with an extra set of keys and scold me and tell me to come home and rest. Sometimes I would, and sometimes not.

Lynne understood that it was her job to keep our home running smoothly and to help me when she could. We were a team.

Things got to the point where St. Norbert, where I grew up was evacuated and the army went in to patrol what was now a ghost town behind high temporary dikes. I remember taking my son with me to tour St. Norbert. Only authorized personnel were allowed in, but I had some pull and I wanted David to see this.

We drove through an empty subdivision larger than most towns, past soldiers in jeeps and stood on top of the south dike which was on top of a street (if you were on the south side of the street, you were out of luck).

We stared out at an inland sea that extended over one hundred miles to the south, past the US border, past Grand Forks to somewhere north of Fargo, North Dakota. Large breakers crashed against the dike. In some areas old school buses where immersed in front of the dike to break the waves and prevent erosion.

We had unusual latitude to resolve problems quickly during this emergency. We just did what we had to do. I remember getting a call from one of the supervisors who reported to me (Eddy Hupalo) in the middle of the night.

It turned out that a dike in a low area of St. Vital in south Winnipeg straddled a septic field, and water was pouring back through the field into the septic tank and then flooding the area. I said, "Get a concrete truck and a pump and fill the tank with the same concrete they use for bridge piers. That will seal the tank."

Eddy said, "We can do that? What about the residents?" I said, "They have to move, tonight. They'd have to move anyway. Knock on their door and give them a heads-up."

And that's how the largest boat anchor in St. Vital was created. Unfortunately, the boys got a little carried away with the concrete and filled all the drains and toilets in the home's basement. It cost us a fair bit of money to sort that one out, but the owners didn't mind. Their house was dry.

There were a lot of heroes from all levels of government and the private sector during that flood. They all made incredible contributions towards fighting the flood. My efforts were quite modest by comparison.

And so it was that through this huge, coordinated effort we fought the one-hundred-year-flood, and we won. But maybe there were other factors as well. I remember walking a deserted street in south Winnipeg one sunny afternoon and looking down through a drain in the street to see water about twelve inches below.

The river had backed up into the land drainage system and was almost at street level. One more severe rain and the flood would have beaten us. It was the Universe that decided to spare Winnipeg, not us mere mortals.

After the flood I authorized a study to establish the extent of hazards in our drainage system like the one that had taken poor Adam. We had no budget for the work. I didn't care. It was going to happen.

We completed the survey and determined that it would take several million dollars over about a year to correct all of the problems. My bosses were totally supportive and the initiative was immediately funded and assigned a high priority. We notified the public of the potential hazards and got to work. In the end we had a safer city, Adam's legacy to us all.

Of course, after the grief, Adam's father became very angry. He called for an inquest and filed a law suit. This resulted in long hours of testimony for me, often with gruelling cross-examination by the plaintiff's lawyer and the judge presiding over the inquest.

It was a media circus and I was at the center of the ring. Some folks at the city were quite indignant that Adam's father took these steps. I wasn't. I understood completely. I would have done the same thing. I would have wanted someone's blood.

In the end, the inquest determined that the City could not have reasonably foreseen the hazard and had taken extraordinary measures to mitigate future events. My conscience was clear. The hazards had been created before my watch, and I had made damn certain that it wouldn't happen again.

The law suit was settled and the amount remains confidential to this day. I hope that Adam's father got a bundle. Adam still haunts me.

The date of Adam's death remained on my calendar for the rest of my working career, a reminder that as an engineer my first duty is to the safety of the public. It is a responsibility that we should all take very seriously.

Lynne stood behind me all through this. She monitored the media and knew when I was being pilloried by one of the local radio talk show vultures. Lynne would tell me, "I know that you are grieving for Adam. You wouldn't be the man I love if you didn't. But it wasn't your fault, and you did all that you could do." I hoped that she was right.

Lynne screened the media calls that I received at all hours, pleasantly telling them that I wasn't available. "When might he be available?" they would ask. She would respond pleasantly that I did not accept calls of this nature at home. Some of them became quite aggressive, and Lynne dispensed with them with a quick wit and a razor tongue. My girl had my back.

That year Lynne turned fifty. I remembered how sensitive she was about our age difference. I thought about it and thought about it.

And then I wrote this poem for her. Lynne loved it. I found it in her jewellery box after she passed on and I remembered her smile when she read it.

The Soul of a Child

*We all have in us
A small part that
Lets us feel and laugh
And Love and think
And look with wonder at the world
Without worry or fear.*

*That part is our youth;
The soul of a child.
And if we protect it
And nurture it
And listen when it speaks,
We will never be old...*

It is no small irony that when Lynne finally passed on, she very much had the soul of a child...

Eventually things got back to normal. And then about a year and a half later something happened that should have destroyed our world and brought us to our knees. But it didn't. All because of the very courageous woman that I married. I am certain that you have heard the hymn *Amazing Grace*. I discovered that I was married to a woman who embodied amazing grace.

Our World Collapses

In early 1999 Lynne and I vacationed on the Gulf Coast in Florida. There was nothing unusual about that. Our favourite places on the planet were the Gulf Coast and Indian Wells, California, where we had a time-share.

As usual, I drove and Lynne navigated. But she missed a lot of turns, which resulted in a few detours and a bit of frustration on my part. In retrospect, this was unusual. Lynne was very good at reading maps, and she never missed anything. I let it pass, we had a nice vacation and we returned home.

After we arrived back home just before Lynne's fifty-first birthday, Lynne told me something that almost caused my heart to stop—and to break. Lynne had always looked after all of our finances and she said, "I can't do this anymore. The numbers just confuse me. I believe that I have Alzheimer's disease."

I said, "That's impossible. You're only fifty years old!" But Lynne had done her research. After six months of testing the doctors confirmed Lynne's diagnosis. As usual, Lynne was right. She had a rare version known as Early On-set Alzheimer's disease.

That's when I truly saw what Lynne was made of. Lynne already knew all about Alzheimer's disease. She always did her homework and she understood fully the terrible future that she faced. After the doctor's diagnosis she looked me in the eye and said, "What will we do?" I said that I would look after her, to which she said, "To the end?" I said yes, that was my promise to her.

Lynne then very methodically made lists of things that I needed to do to carry on family traditions: birthday lists, menus for Christmas, and so on. Then she prompted me to arrange for her will, power of attorney and health care directive.

And we got on with our lives. Lynne didn't want Alzheimer's to define her and she didn't want to talk about it. Not once did I see Lynne despair or feel sorry for herself. Her courage and grace astounded me.

It was then that I made a vow to myself. I vowed that I would do whatever was required to keep my beautiful, brave wife safe and happy and loved, until she left this earth. And as Lynne would tell you, I have many faults, but I always keep my promises.

Life changes

A couple of things fell into place for me after the doctors confirmed Lynne's diagnosis. We had purchased a new car the fall prior (a sporty little Cougar, fully loaded. Back then, we were a Ford family) and despite my urging Lynne had never driven it. She said she preferred the comfort of her Mercury. I realized then that the reason she had not driven it was that she couldn't figure out the buttons in the car.

I also realized why Lynne had so much trouble navigating in Florida and I was very sad that I had been impatient with her. I told her that, and she simply said, "Tom, it's OK. There is no way that you could have known. I know that you love me." That just made me feel worse.

Lynne had always managed our household, paid the bills and made the investments. She was very good at it and it is because of her that we were able to sustain the lifestyle we had. I doubt that I would have been able to retire at the age of fifty-nine without Lynne at the helm for most of our married life. So I didn't meddle.

The money went into the bank and Lynne worked her magic. If I wanted to make a major purchase (like a new car), I talked to Lynne and she told me whether we could afford one. We always made decisions as a team, and if we disagreed we would talk it through until we were both satisfied. There were no arguments about money in our household.

Once Lynne told me that she thought she had Alzheimer's disease it became my responsibility to handle the household finances. This may seem like a small thing. Many men do it. However, I had quite a learning curve.

The accounts were in disarray and several bills were past due. I didn't even know what bills came in every month or whether Lynne had them set up for automatic payment or whether I had to cut a check. Whenever I called to explain to someone why they hadn't been paid, they were very understanding. I think that most people just want to do the right thing.

After a couple of months I had done my forensic sleuthing and had a system set up that almost looked after itself. I knew that all my spare time was going to be taken up caring for Lynne and I didn't want to worry about bills. I also knew that I needed to marshal resources for Lynne's care. It was going to be a long, expensive ride.

The other thing that happened immediately after Lynne's diagnosis was that she lost her driver's licence. Apparently, for public safety reasons that is standard procedure when a diagnosis of cognitive impairment is rendered.

This upset Lynne greatly. Her freedom had been taken from her. I can recall her riding along with me, pointing at some errant driver and ranting, "Look at that bozo! And they won't let *me* drive!"

Interestingly, after Lynne began taking a drug called Aricept, she improved so much that her doctor said that she could re-apply for her licence. Sadly, Lynne knew that this would be only a temporary respite and she decided that she had more important ways to spend her time.

Lynne's doctor was a gentleman named Dr. Barry Campbell. I say gentleman, because that is exactly what he was. He had a kind gentle demeanour and he treated both Lynne and me with empathy and respect. Often as part of our visits Dr. Campbell needed to administer a mini-mental test to gauge the rate of Lynne's decline. These caused Lynne a great deal of stress and she became very upset when she couldn't answer some of the test questions. She knew that she had lost so much.

Dr. Campbell always patiently helped Lynne through it. He prescribed Aricept for Lynne. This drug can offer some temporary improvement to some people with Alzheimer's when initially administered, and slow the rate of progression of the disease. It does not work for everyone, and an early diagnosis is paramount.

For Lynne it was a wonder drug, and it enhanced the quality of both our lives for several years. At the time, our health care system did not cover the drug and it was very costly. I didn't care. For Lynne and me it was priceless. It gave me a few more years with my girl.

During our first visit, even before the diagnosis Dr. Campbell urged us to get our affairs in order. This meant wills, powers of attorney and health care directives. Lynne had already thought of this, but my mind was focused on other things and I simply procrastinated.

After our visit to Dr. Campbell, Lynne hounded me relentlessly until I made the necessary arrangements. I discovered that the wife of a retired colleague (Carole Hreno) practised law from her home. This kind, patient woman prepared the necessary documents and prompted both Lynne and me through their execution with minimal stress.

A word of caution: *It is very important that these documents are executed while the patient is still competent and able to sign. Alzheimer's will fairly quickly cause some people to lose the ability to sign their own name. In the absence of these authorities banks have been known to freeze assets, leaving caregivers with no resources. Bankers aren't bad people, but they are bound by the law and operate by their own peculiar set of rules, which leave little room for empathy or common sense.*

Lynne had many family customs that she valued greatly and she didn't want them lost. She made lists of Christmas and New Year's menus, and other favourites of Dave's and mine. We continued to follow all of our family traditions.

David and I would decorate the tree with Lynne watching us raptly. We always got about a twelve foot tree, and stood it up next to the stair landing in the living room so that we could reach the top without a ladder. When Dave was little I used to hold him out and he would place the ornaments. By the time Lynne that got sick, these roles were reversed, and Dave hung onto me while I leant over to decorate the tree.

We baked Lynne's signature shortbread. The first year, Lynne participated although Dave was the brains behind the operation. (Lynne taught him to bake at an early age). Later, she was happy to watch and smile.

When Dave asked her what was up with the lists, Lynne responded kindly that the time would soon come when she would be unable to remember these things and gave him a hug. No tears. No drama. Just bravery and grace.

I know how distressed Dave must have been about his mom, but he put on a good face. Dave stepped up and became Mom's taxi when I wasn't available. He took her grocery shopping for as long as she was able to manage that. He must have felt a lot of pressure. He had just started university that fall.

For my part, I held back the tears while I was in front of Lynne or David, but I spent a lot of time in the garage, crying.

For the first couple of years Lynne was safe at home alone. This is actually quite unusual for people with dementia, and I think that the Aricept helped in that regard. I set up an office in our guest room and worked a couple of days a week from home, via a secure internet link set up by our IT staff and by telephone.

I would go to the office about three days a week to attend meetings and deal with staff on a face-to-face basis. Lynne was still pretty smart. She would not answer the door if I wasn't home, and she would not leave the house. Lynne didn't want to get lost.

As an aside: *Many people with Alzheimer's wander and this is a significant personal safety concern. Some form of wristband with the person's name, address and caregiver's contact information is a very good idea. They now have wristbands that can be tracked by radio frequency. A huge step forward!*

Lynne almost immediately lost the ability to operate the TV remote, and dial the telephone. I put my office and cell phones on speed-dial (green button for office and red for cell phone) and left instructions with my assistant Rose to interrupt me whenever Lynne called. No matter what.

Lynne had always made sure that we had a nice gift and a card for Rose at Christmas. Rose is a good hearted woman and she would chat with Lynne while she tenaciously hunted me down. My cell phone which used to remain off during meetings was now on at all times. I didn't care who I interrupted. No one was as important as Lynne.

After many telephone calls from Lynne to talk her through how to change TV stations I sat down with her and we talked about what shows she liked. I was able to program the TV to change channels automatically and this helped a lot.

Lynne and I were still able to live a reasonable life back then. We continued to travel for vacations and to board meetings, but I curtailed all other business travel and volunteer work. I had another more important priority—my wife's care and happiness.

The folks at the board meetings were always very good to Lynne and many wives asked if they could spend some time with Lynne, to keep her company. But Lynne didn't seem to feel safe with anyone but me, so she would politely decline and spend her time in the room when I was in meetings.

I would wait for an opportune time on the agenda and go up to the room to check on her and bring her a snack. Yogurt and a muffin always brought a smile to her face.

We did go to one last conference in Atlanta, Georgia in in June, 2002. We stayed in the Westin tower downtown, and it was a memorable trip for several reasons. We took a cab from the airport and as we waited in line to check in I realized that Lynne had left her purse in the taxi.

All of our credit cards, ID and passports were in the purse. I tried to explain the situation to the desk clerk, even telling her that Lynne suffered from Alzheimer's disease, but she wouldn't let us check in. Lynne was in tears. She thought that it was all her fault. Of course it wasn't. It was my stupidity for not keeping tabs on the purse.

I was just in between consoling Lynne and checking my wallet to see if I had enough cash to check in when a voice behind me, a fellow Canadian who was a total stranger said, "Here. Put it on *my* card. He can square up with me later." He gave me a business card and I thanked him profusely. He brushed it off as common courtesy. What a wonderful, kind gesture!

We checked in and I quickly went down to the taxi stand and gave the bell captain a description of the cab and the driver. I asked him to ask the driver to wait if he located him, and said that I would come down and retrieve the purse. The bell captain bounded off down the street like a gazelle in pursuit of the cab. He recognized the description of the driver and thought that he knew where the driver might wait for his next fare.

I went up to the room to wait with Lynne, who by now had calmed down a bit. Twenty minutes later there was a knock on the door and there was the bell captain with the purse, with contents intact. I gave him fifty dollars and asked him if the driver was still downstairs.

He said, "Yes, the driver is there." I went downstairs to thank the driver personally and to give him fifty dollars as well. By the way, he was an African American with Rasta dreadlocks, which had inspired some trepidation in Lynne. But he was a good, honest man. *Books and covers...*

Security was very tight at the Westin. It was the summer after nine-eleven and the Westin was the tallest building in Atlanta. You needed to be a registered guest and have ID just to get in and out of the place, and to board the elevators. This made quite an impression on Lynne.

I still remember Lynne's reaction when she heard the news about nine-eleven. She was in the very early stages of

Alzheimer's and she understood fully what had happened. She called me on my cell phone to tell me about it, in tears.

Her last words were, "I hope that bastard Bin Laden roasts in hell!" Those were very strong words for Lynne. Lynne would have liked President Obama for a lot of reasons, but bringing Bin Laden to justice would have been at the top of the list.

Incidentally, she didn't have a lot of use for George Bush, also for a lot of reasons, not the least of which were his policies on abortion and stem cell research (which offers hope of a cure for many diseases, including Alzheimer's disease).

Lynne was a strong advocate of women's rights and the disenfranchised. Before and after she had Alzheimer's disease, she used to giggle helplessly any time there was someone doing a parody of President Bush on Letterman or SNL.

The mention of giggles recalls the other highpoint of our Atlanta trip. Lynne was a big fan of *Gone with the Wind*, and she wanted to go to Miss Pitty Pat's Porch across the street for dinner. Which we did. It was wonderful, even if my cholesterol spiked into the stratosphere!

Before we went, we decided to go to the revolving bar at the top of the Westin for a drink. About half way, up a well-known African American comedian (it may have been Chris Rock) boarded the elevator, along with a retinue that included a big hefty guy (I'm guessing a body guard), some very attractive women and a couple of buddies.

He looked at us, two past-middle-aged white folks, dressed in jeans and white sneakers and said, "Where you two goin? Y'all goin to the sock hop?" His delivery was impeccable and it was obvious that he wasn't insulting us. He was just being his very funny self. Lynne started to laugh uncontrollably and finally said, "I'm sorry, I can't help it! I have Alzheimer's Disease." The comedian got off the elevator with a very perplexed look on his face.

I attended an Alzheimer Care Givers support group throughout Lynne's illness. Initially, I resisted. I wasn't much of a "group" person and most of the group members were much older than me. I am so glad I changed my mind.

These people became a second family to me. We shared our experiences and we shared our grief every month. We were all looking after loved ones at different stages of the disease and we were able to provide helpful advice, solace and contacts.

There was also a support group for people with dementia, but Lynne would not have anything to do with it. She just wanted to live her life and spend time with me, knowing that I loved her and that she loved me.

So we lived our lives. Every weekend for breakfast, I would take Lynne to the Forks (a trendy area at the confluence of the Red and Assiniboine Rivers). Lynne always had French toast and blueberries, which we shared. We would then walk down the way and buy a couple of date cookies and coffee. Lynne liked them and she said that they were almost as good as the ones she used to make.

We would often walk along the river walk at the Forks or around the lakes near our home. Interestingly, when we got close to home Lynne would always turn up the driveway next to ours. That is where her best friend Shirley lived until she moved away, and I think that part of Lynne yearned for her friend.

Alzheimer's disease isolates you. People don't know what to say and all but the most dedicated friends stop coming around. Lynne's lifelong friend Irene would come to visit, but I think that Lynne was embarrassed about her loss of abilities, so it was awkward for Lynne and emotionally devastating for Irene. Irene still kept coming, for long as she was able to. Eventually it was just too hard on her.

Lynne was always very particular about her personal hygiene and grooming. After a while she began to forget steps and she asked be to make up some laminated cards which listed the steps that she needed to take. With the cards, she was able to get ready in the mornings on her own for quite a while, over three years.

Sadly though, after about three and a half years Lynne lost the ability to read anything complex, and the ability to write. This was a great loss to her because she had always been an avid reader. She devoured the newspaper and several current-affairs magazines on a weekly basis before she became ill. I always received the daily news and a current affairs update in a succinct summary from Lynne at our dinner table!

Lynne always had her hair done by a stylist named Harold, who at that time was working out of his home on Arlington Street. Lynne had actually been going to see Harold for longer than she had known me.

I used to take a morning off work when Lynne needed a cut and a colour (about once a month) and off we would go to visit Harold. I would wait for Lynne to get her "do" and listen to Harold tell Lynne dirty jokes. He would soon have her in stitches. He seemed to be the only person besides me who could get Lynne to laugh at that time.

I know that the news of Lynne's illness was devastating to Harold, but he never let it show in front of Lynne. He only wanted to make her laugh. I'll tell you a little more about Harold later in this book and about a dental hygienist named Cheryl who also helped Lynne.

And so it was that until this point in time, the Universe had conspired through the kindness of both friends and strangers to help Lynne and me along our way. But remember what I said. Sometimes the Universe works in strange ways, and nothing was going to prepare me for what happened next.

Divine Intervention

Two summers after Lynne's diagnosis, right after we returned from Atlanta, we were combining a little business and pleasure. It was Saturday morning and I had just taken Lynne for breakfast at the Forks, and we went for a short walk along the river afterwards. It was a beautiful, sunny summer day.

My plan was to stop by a water main repair on the way home. There had been a large break in Portage Avenue and it had shut down all of the westbound lanes during rush-hour. It made the Friday evening news and the front page of the Saturday paper and I wanted to make sure that our crew had it under control and that traffic would at least be semi-restored by Monday.

I didn't feel well. Initially I put it off to indigestion, but after we visited the repair I could feel a pressure in my chest, and my anxiety began to build. I didn't want to alarm Lynne, so I said very casually that I was going to stop by the Victoria Hospital because I had indigestion and I wanted them to check me out. By this time, Lynne's condition had progressed to the point where she didn't grasp the import of what I had said.

I pulled into the emergency bay at the hospital and we went inside. I described my condition to the triage nurse and she said, "You have to go back there. Now!" She turned to Lynne and said, "You have to move that car. It's in the way!" Lynne said, "Oh no. I can't drive. I have Alzheimer's disease!"

Did I mention that they have valet parking at the Victoria Hospital? I handed the keys to the nurse and she got a candy striper to move our sporty little Cougar. When the young girl returned, she said, "That's a nice little car!" The things you remember...

Anyway, they put me in a gown and hooked me up to monitors while the young girl sat and kept Lynne company. They tried to contact my son Dave, to no avail. Finally I called my neighbour Larry and asked him to go over and pound on the door. It turned out that Dave had succumbed to a migraine headache and was sleeping with the phones turned off.

Dave came down to the hospital in our second car with a friend to pick up Lynne and take our car home.

In the meantime the Docs were running a battery of tests. They decreed that I had not had a heart attack, but things weren't right and I needed an angiogram to assess my condition. At this point I was more worried about Lynne than myself. I asked if they could send Dave and Lynne in to talk to me.

I told Lynne that I needed to stay in the hospital for a while so they could figure out what was wrong me. I said it was no big deal, but by then Lynne was on to me. She looked at Dave and rolled her eyes! I said that we needed to ask someone to come and help her out while I was in the hospital, and we could either ask her sister-in-law (Jack's wife) or my sister Lynn.

Lynne said that she would prefer my sister Lynn, so I made the call and she was there the next day, from northern Alberta. I covered the airfare.

The three of them visited every day. After a few days they shipped me over the cardiac center at St. Boniface Hospital where I was told that they would do the angiogram. If things looked good they would install stents then and there. If not, they would discuss my prognosis.

Getting an angiogram was a unique experience. We were lined up on stretchers like cars going through a car wash. One patient would be going in as another was leaving! Modern medicine!

Anyway, they inject a dye and you could watch the progress of a probe on a screen as they push the probe through your blood vessels to your heart. I joked with the nurse that it was a little like sewer televising! *Yes, we do send cameras down sewers to assess their condition.* She looked at me as though I had lost my mind.

The doctor came in and told me very succinctly (I'm guessing it took maybe a minute) that I was not a candidate for stents, that I had four very severe blockages and that I would require open-heart by-pass surgery. And then out I went to recovery. No fuss, no muss.

As I lay in recovery I tried to process what the Doc had told me. I needed open heart surgery. I was terrified that I wouldn't make it. Not because I was afraid to die. I needed to be there to look after my Lynne.

I have never been particularly religious. After I met Lynne, I pulled up my socks and lived a better life. I was faithful. I tried to see the best in people and help them. I tried to be a good husband and father. But I never went to church, except for weddings and funerals.

Nonetheless, I closed my eyes and I prayed. I prayed that God would spare me so that I could care for Lynne until God took her. And I prayed for strength and compassion, so that I could properly fulfill that obligation; that duty borne out of love. Nevertheless, I remember thinking how unfair it was that this trial was being visited upon me. It turned out that I was wrong about that.

They shipped me back to the Victoria Hospital to wait for a consultation with a surgeon. As the ambulance bounced along Winnipeg's streets (I think that Winnipeg must be the pothole capital of Canada!), I thought about how I was going to break the news to Lynne and David.

When I explained the outcome to Lynne, I know that she was as afraid as I was, but she didn't show it. All Lynne showed me was love and concern. Years later, my sister told me a few things about Lynne's actions while I was in the hospital.

Lynne always had a couple of stories for me when she visited. Apparently, she would read the paper, looking for items that she thought I would be interested in, and then tell them to Dave and my sister, so they could prompt her to tell the story if she forgot.

Once on the way to the hospital, Dave wasn't paying attention and he rear-ended another car. Lynne didn't care a bit about the damage to our car, but she did say very sternly to Dave and my sister, "Tom doesn't need to hear about this. He shouldn't be exposed to any stress!"

My dear Lynne was looking after me even then.

I spent about two weeks in the emergency ward before they found me a room on the fifth floor. During that time some of the nurses came to chat. One night one of them came to do a check of my vital signs, and then sat on the edge of the bed and we talked.

She said that she had heard that my wife had Alzheimer's disease and that it must be very difficult. Then she said that she had seen many cases where a spouse just walked away in similar situations.

I said, "Lynne has looked after me for almost twenty-five years. Now it is my turn to look after her." She said, "It will be very, very hard." To which I replied, "Lynne loves me with all of her heart. And I love her. I will do whatever needs to be done." The nurse replied, "Just don't die trying." And then she left.

There was a shortage of cardiac surgeons back then and the waits for surgery were very long. My GP was a nice guy and he told me not to under any circumstances agree to be discharged, or I would wait another six months for surgery. He told me to have them call him if there was any hint that they were trying to discharge me.

After a few more days, I was sent over to meet the surgeon. I was sent by ambulance. Lynne and David met me there and sat with me while I waited. It was a very long wait and I was getting annoyed because I thought that it must be hard for Lynne and it was very tiring for me.

Finally, it was our turn. It was an interesting session. The surgeon explained what was necessary to do the by-pass. I asked him whether there were other options. He said yes, you could forego the surgery, and you would die.

I was more than a little pissed that he said that in front of Lynne. He went on to say that I seemed to be doing well and that he was going to send me home from his office to await surgery there. *Aha. The end run.*

I went back into the waiting room where I became so agitated that I experienced chest pains. Not good for business if you're a vascular surgeon! The nurse called an ambulance and they stabilized me and took me back to the Victoria Hospital where I waited another four weeks before surgery. In my mind, my surgeon was an arrogant young Prima Donna. I didn't like him at all. But he got the job done, eventually.

During the four more weeks I spent at the Victoria Hospital my sister or Dave (or both) would bring Lynne to visit. I discovered later that there had been some fireworks between Lynne and my sister, but Lynne never said a word in front of me. She would rather endure what amounted to abuse than subject me to stress.

Much later, after Lynne's death I learned that there were times when my sister essentially treated Lynne like a child, withholding food privileges when they disagreed. My sister spent a long time away from home while caring for Lynne while I was hospitalized. I am indebted to her for that, but I will never forgive that behaviour. I doubt that my son will either.

After what seemed like forever to me, a nurse came in and said that I was scheduled for surgery at the Health Sciences Centre and would be transferred by ambulance the next day. The surgery would be performed the day after the transfer at four a.m.

Of course, Lynne and David wanted to come and see me at that early hour, before I went into the operating room. I said, "No." The Health Sciences Centre is located in the core area of Winnipeg and it is a long walk from parking to the hospital. It wasn't safe. There was some disagreement between us about this, but eventually they relented.

I was transferred to Health Sciences Centre and they woke me up around three a.m. the next day and prepped me for surgery. I felt very alone. Then the call came in. There had been a terrible car accident and one of the survivors needed major surgery or they wouldn't live. I was bumped.

Later in the day, my surgeon came in and said that he could perform the surgery the next day, if I didn't mind being moved to St. Boniface Hospital. I said, "Sure, let's get it done." So they moved me that day, and my surgery was scheduled for five a.m. the next morning.

St. Boniface Hospital is in a much better part of town, and after feeling so very alone I truly wanted my family present when I went into surgery. And so it was that the last thing I saw before I went into surgery were two pairs of loving, concerned brown eyes looking down at me. My wife and my son. Lynne walked along the gurney, clinging to my hand right up to the operating room door.

I remember waking up after the surgery and hearing sounds before I opened my eyes and thinking *Hmm. I guess I made it!* That thought was followed by feelings of intense joy, relief and pain.

The pain eventually subsided, but the joy and relief remained. I made it! I would be there for Lynne! Lynne and David were eventually allowed to see me, albeit only briefly. Lynne looked worried but happy. Dave was very quiet. I think that he was worried too.

They don't keep you in the hospital very long after bypass surgery anymore. I was there for about five days, which is longer than the norm. The main reasons that my stay was longer had to do with the logistics of setting up home care for me, and home care for Lynne.

I would be too weak initially to care for myself and Lynne couldn't do it. I couldn't look after Lynne either, so she needed homecare. For reasons that to this day elude me, the arrangements could not be made by the hospital social worker.

The hospital social worker made my arrangements and a social worker in the community made Lynne's. It took a while for them to coordinate. The other reason was pretty simple. Once the home care fell into place, we were into a long weekend, and the Doc and whomever else were needed to sign off on the discharge were not around.

Anyway, they eventually turned me loose and my sister, Lynne and David came to pick me up. I was instructed firmly by the nurse to ride in the back seat of the car with a pillow between the seatbelt and my chest to protect the incision. I think that I was supposed to do that for about a month.

Apparently if you were up front and an airbag went off, things could get nasty if the bone where the chest was cut opened had not healed. Lynne often forgot things by that time. Her short term memory was going. But she remembered that edict and enforced it strictly! She wasn't about to let anything bad happen to her Tom!

My sister left shortly after I returned home, and Lynne, David and I were on our own again. David would be in classes during the day and he was out many evenings, so Lynne and I were on our own except when home care came in to check on us.

Lynne would hover around me and ask me over and over again if I was OK. She was concerned about me and because of the Alzheimer's she would forget that she had asked me the same question five minutes ago. I didn't mind! I was ecstatic to be home with Lynne and I felt very, very loved.

Lynne would give me hugs, but she approached the problem as though she was hugging a porcupine! She was afraid that she would hurt me.

I was told that I was not supposed to lift anything at all initially, and wasn't allowed to drive for six weeks. We had a two story home, and I had to be careful on the stairs. Too much exertion made me dizzy. At first, I had to climb to the landing, rest a bit and then finish the climb.

Lynne would be at my elbow, waiting to steady me if I wobbled. Often I would awake from a nap to find her sitting by the bed watching me intently. Then she would give me a blinding smile. We were both very happy to be together again!

As you already know, Lynne could not drive, so for the first six weeks David or one of my friends would chauffeur me to my medical appointments. Lynne would come along because by this time I wasn't comfortable leaving her alone.

My co-workers on the management team at work generously arranged for catered dinners to be delivered to our home for about a month. They knew that Lynne couldn't cook anymore, and I wasn't able to.

One other meal was delivered during that period. This one resulted in a funny reaction from one of my neighbours! Another co-worker named Phil Lee called and wanted to bring me some Chinese food. At the time, in addition to working at the City, Phil and his family owned a couple of Chinese restaurants. Phil was quite successful.

He assured me that the food would be prepared under his supervision and that it would not violate any of the dietary restrictions that my Docs had imposed upon me. I was touched by Phil's generosity. I assumed that Phil would have the food delivered by his staff so I was even more touched when he turned up at our door himself.

But here is the funny part. Picture your neighbour out cutting his grass when someone delivers Chinese food. Except that the delivery guy is wearing a thousand dollar suit with an Order of Canada pin (a great honour, by the way) on his lapel and driving a shiny new very expensive Lexus!

Lynne was watching all this from the front window and she started to giggle when she saw the expression on my neighbour's face! So Phil brought us a lovely dinner and some entertainment as well. Phil has always worked diligently for the community and has generously donated enormous amounts of time to various efforts. He is now retired from the city, but he was appointed Lieutenant Governor of Manitoba a while back; another great honour that keeps him very busy.

After six weeks I had recovered to the point where I could walk around the bay where we lived. Lynne would always be waiting anxiously at the door when I returned. Once I could drive again I started to attend a cardiac rehab program.

Lynne attended some of the lifestyle classes with me, but I think that she found it a bit confusing. I resumed taking her to her scheduled visits with Dr. Campbell, and we went for breakfast at the Forks twice weekly, and walked afterwards. And the calls began. When was I coming back to work?

I loved my job, but it was very demanding and quite stressful. I had just fewer than three hundred folks working for me at the time, and there were always a few bad apples to deal with. Just before being hospitalized for my surgery I had attended a very acrimonious appeal hearing associated with a staff member that I had dismissed.

The hearing was chaired by a neutral lawyer who would rule on whether dismissal would be upheld or whether the Union's appeal would succeed. There was legal counsel present from both sides, and I had to testify. The employee had alleged ties to a biker gang and I had recommended dismissal because he had threatened a supervisor.

During my recovery period the Chair rendered his decision and the employee was dismissed. A few days later I opened the garage door to back the car out and our driveway was covered with shingle nails. I swept them up and went in and thought long and hard about what to do. I did not tell Lynne about the incident. She protected me, and I protected her. She did not need the worry.

I talked to my doctor about the incident and my work. He said that if Lynne were healthy he thought that I would be OK to return to my job, but that I would need to keep my hours at around forty a week, not the fifty plus that I had been working.

He then told me that if I was caring for Lynne and doing my job I would almost certainly end up back in the hospital. That made up my mind. I loved my wife a lot more than my work.

I met with our human resources manager, Angie Munch. Angie and I had faced many issues together (including the most recent dismissal) and she wasn't just a co-worker. She was a very good friend with my best interests at heart.

She understood what I was going through and her advice was to stay home, remain on sick leave and apply for a disability pension. This would require my doctor's support and would need to be authorized by the City's Employee Benefits Board. I took Angie's advice and as a result I was able to stay home and care for Lynne for three years. I was very relieved and happy.

Remember when I said that the Universe works in strange ways? I had heart problems that left untreated could have resulted in a fatal heart attack. But they didn't. I got a warning bout of sever angina (no heart attack) and received the necessary surgery to correct the problem.

And then I was afforded the opportunity to bail on my stressful job and care for Lynne full-time! What I had originally considered as a terrible adversity had turned out to be an incredible gift.

The Universe continued to watch over Lynne and me, and I had much to be thankful for. And I thanked God for my good fortune.

Making the most of the time we have

My recovery from by-pass surgery went very well, and before long I was able to work out at the cardiac rehab center and became stronger and healthier by the day. I spent the rest of my time with Lynne, just doing the things that you need to do from day to day; helping her get dressed in the morning, shopping for groceries and making meals.

By then I had a house-keeper (Katie) who came in once a week to clean. Lynne and I usually went out to the Forks for breakfast while Katie cleaned. I had a service that did yard maintenance in the summer and another that did our snow clearing in the winter. My focus was on Lynne, and making her life as happy and full as I possibly could.

Lynne loved to travel, and even then she enjoyed new scenery and particularly walks. She enjoyed walks on the beach and she enjoyed walks in the moonlight near our time-share in Indian Wells. The clear skies at night in Indian Wells against the outline of the Santa Rosa Mountains during a full moon were magic to her.

Travelling was complicated for Lynne and she did best in a consistent environment. So I bought a thirty-five foot motor home and a new Honda Accord to tow behind it, and this became our freedom machine. Every October we would load up the RV, hitch the car up behind it and off we would go for about six weeks.

We would take a different route each year and head down to Padre Island, Texas over about a two week period. Then we would spend three or four weeks on the beach before heading back for Christmas. The last few days heading back were timed to coincide with good driving conditions, and it was "pedal–to-the-metal" once the temperature went below freezing.

We toured South Dakota and Colorado. Once, we went through west Texas and followed the Rio Grande down to the gulf. While we were driving through west Texas there was not a lot on the radio except for country-western music.

Neither one of us was a big fan of this genre, but we would sing along—and Lynne would laugh until her tummy ached!

Sedona, Santa Fe and San Antonio were favourites for Lynne. She particularly enjoyed San Antonio. She had already been there many times with me for business conferences and Lynne loved the River Walk. We visited a feisty Texan named Kay Kutchins while we were there. Kay and I had served on a board together and she made it her mission to ensure that we saw the best that San Antonio had to offer. She was a very gracious host and she doted on Lynne.

While we were on Padre Island we stayed in a campground on the beach. It had full hook-ups (power, sewer and water and cable TV) so it was like being at home. Lynne loved our walks on the beach, with the sun beating down and the salt spray in the air. Even though it was November, the temperature was about perfect for us snow-birds.

We went to a fish shop owned by a Hispanic family to buy fresh fish and shrimp, which I barbequed for dinner as we dined outside at the picnic table. The Hispanic family could tell that something wasn't quite right with Lynne. When I confided to the owner that Lynne had Alzheimer's disease his eyes filled with tears, and he said that they would pray for her. After that his wife always greeted Lynne with a hug.

In March of 2005 Lynne and I spent a week at our time share in Indian Wells. We had been to the time share many times and Lynne was very comfortable there. We did our treasured walk in the moonlight and I barbequed fresh fish for us every night.

Lynne was doing pretty well on that trip, so we drove up to Monterey and spent a couple of days there before flying back to Winnipeg. There were lots of things to see and do in Monterey—good restaurants and good scenery.

I attended my last winter board meeting during the spring after we bought the RV. It was in San Juan, Puerto

Rico and we added an extra week to the trip so that we could see the island. We had a great time, but the meetings were hard on Lynne, as she spent long stretches alone in our room.

I was an officer on the board and that meant that I pretty much had to stay in the meeting during the formal agenda to present the budget and respond to questions from the other board members. I was about half-way through my term as treasurer and it had been a great achievement to be appointed as an officer in the organization. There had been only one other Canadian in the history of the organization to have served in such a senior capacity.

After the meetings over a dinner of tapas I could see that the hours in the room had worn on Lynne. So I said, "Are you looking forward to touring the island?" Lynne said, "Yes, very much. It will just be you and me."

I said to her, "I'm tired of sharing my time on these trips with other people. I am resigning from the board after we return home. From now on it's just you and me all the time, kiddo!" Lynne gave me a brilliant smile, a smile that I still hold in my heart today.

After that, we were tourists. We toured old San Juan. We toured the Bacardi distillery (a favourite of mine!) We went to the beach. We went to El Yunque rain forest. We had a wonderful week.

Two things of significance occurred over the next two years. Lynne started to deteriorate more quickly, and the pressure for me to reengage in work began to build.

As Lynne's cognitive abilities began to decline, she became easily disoriented and I had to keep a close eye on her to make sure that she didn't get lost. I received an award from a professional organization (the American Water Works Association) in June of 2005 and I had to attend the annual conference in San Francisco to receive it.

It was a big deal. The award was for service to the water industry and only one of the fifty-five thousand members is given the award each year. I was the second Canadian to have ever received the award and Lynne was very proud of me.

The award was delivered on-stage at the opening session by the American Water Works Association president. Lots of hoopla. Because of my worries about Lynne, I asked two co-workers who were in attendance to sit with Lynne and help her out. They were both ladies, so if Lynne needed to go to the restroom one could go with her. Everything went well and Lynne sat quietly through the ceremony and was happy to see me receive my award.

I had checked us into the Hyatt at Fisherman's Wharf and immediately after the award we turned into tourists. I had no intention wasting one precious minute at the conference when I could be with Lynne! As I was busy on the wharf buying ferry tickets to Sausalito I turned my head for a second and Lynne wandered off.

I found her a minute later standing in the middle of a crowd, terrified, with tears streaming down her face. Lesson learned. That was the last time Lynne's hand ever left mine when we were out. I would even find family restrooms in the airports, so that I could accompany her if she needed to go.

Our last trip by air was to Florida, and it was a horror story. I booked a large condo on the beach and I guess it was just too big for Lynne. She would get turned around and become afraid unless I was in the room. At night I would have to accompany her to the restroom because she was afraid to go on her own.

I do have two good memories of that trip. One was after I took Lynne to a fairly high end restaurant for dinner as a treat. I asked her if she enjoyed it, and she said, "I'm sorry Tom, but I like your cooking better!" I wasn't upset. I felt complimented!

I knew that Lynne felt stressed by that time when we went to restaurants. She had trouble reading the menus and if I read them to her, she had trouble recalling the selections. Lynne also knew good food when she tasted it and she genuinely enjoyed my cooking. So I pulled out all the stops and we dined like kings every night on our balcony while we watched the sun go down.

The other wonderful memory is of Lynne walking along the beach in the sunshine; strolling through the tidal pools in her sneakers and not caring if her shoes were wet, smiling serenely!

But the trip home was tough. When we cleared security to return home the agent was adamant that I had to stand three feet from Lynne while she was screened, and that she had to stand three feet from me while I was screened. I explained that Lynne had Alzheimer's disease and this would be terrifying for her. He didn't care. Rules are rules.

So Lynne stood by weeping in terror while the screening took place. After he was done, I informed the agent that there was a special place in hell, and it was reserved just for him. The other passengers who witnessed this travesty applauded. Some had other far more pointed remarks for the agent as well.

Finally, at the end of our trip as we were disembarking in Winnipeg, there was no ramp available and Lynne had to descend the steep stairs from the door of the airplane. She lost her balance and fell at the bottom. The airline staff whisked her into a wheelchair and through customs. Lynne was not hurt, but she was distressed and embarrassed. That is when I decided, "No more airplanes for us—we'll stick with the RV."

My case manager at EBB decided that I should start working part-time. I talked to my doctor, who was well aware of Lynne's condition and he said, "No problem as long as it is no more than two days a week, from home." When they pressed him on why I had to work from home he essentially said he was the doctor, and that was his determination.

With technology, it was quite easy for me to work from home with minimal contact with the outside world. Now and then, staff would actually bring me paperwork and attend meetings at our dining room table.

The IT guys came up with an ingenious way for me to work from the RV while Lynne and I travelled. I had a cell phone with a special long distance plan, and a card that I could slip into my laptop to access the internet. So I even worked while I was on the road and I was able to bank a huge amount of vacation time that I knew I was going to need later on for Lynne's care if I had to return to work.

Towards the end of my three years of disability leave my case manager got wind that I was working while I was out of town and he lowered the boom. He said that if you leave Winnipeg while on disability you must take vacation time. He didn't care if I was working while I was away.

He also said that EBB would soon be undertaking an assessment to determine when (not "if") I was to return to work full time. All of this had me pretty worked up. I went to see my doctor and we discussed what was happening. His view was that the only way I would be able to avoid a return to work would be if they took into account how it would affect Lynne. That was not likely to be part of EBB's considerations.

My doctor then suggested that in view of what I was going through, I consider some stress leave before I needed to return to work. Even though I had used six months of sick leave while I was going through by-pass surgery, I still had a huge reserve of leave. I had very seldom missed work due to illness.

I said that the best medicine for me would be one last trip with Lynne in our RV. He said, "How much time would you need?" I said, "Six weeks." My doctor wrote me a note and Lynne and I hit the road one last time. I did not work for one minute while I was gone.

After I returned home the reassessment began. I dragged it out as long as I possibly could. Through various means I was able to buy several more months, but in the end I knew that I had to go back to work. Please understand; it wasn't that I didn't want to work. But Lynne was declining quickly and I was very worried that without me there to stimulate her and keep her company she would get worse even more rapidly. Lynne was my priority.

So I made it as difficult as I could for EBB; I ensured that they understood fully that my return to work would hasten my wife's decline, and asked them point blank if they were really going to force me to do it anyway. Predictably, they said that Lynne's decline was regrettable, but it was not EBB's mandate or concern.

I actually looked carefully at our finances to see whether there were enough reserves to allow me to retire then, but there just wasn't enough money.

So I made arrangements for full-time care for Lynne while I was at work and some respite care in the evenings. My social worker from Manitoba Homecare was a kind, empathic person and she made sure that I had the resources that I needed. And I went back to work.

Back to work and the long road down

By the time I returned to work Alzheimer's disease was taking its toll on Lynne, but she could still have fun. By this time Lynne had long since lost her ability to read and write, to dress herself and to bathe, to brush and floss her teeth and to do her hair. Those were now my responsibilities. I became a manicurist and a hair stylist between visits to Harold.

Yet Lynne still enjoyed going to the Forks for French toast and she loved her birthday parties, with cake and ice cream and candles and a Happy Birthday song!

Two angels from Homecare, Janet and Wendy, looked after Lynne most of the time while I worked. Lynne was not able to speak in complete sentences anymore, so her verbal communication abilities were somewhat limited, but I always knew what she wanted. Her non-verbal skills (a smile, a laugh, a surprised look or a scowl) always filled in the blanks. And thank God, she still recognized me.

About that time, we had to be a lot more selective about what Lynne watched on television. You see, she began to think that what was happening in the TV was real. She would walk up to the TV and pat the screen and gently say, "There, there" when a character was upset. Programs such as CSI were simply too graphic and frightening for her to watch.

Lynne used to be quite the *fashioneesta* when she was well, and once while we were breakfasting at the Forks she spied an outrageously dressed woman (kind of a punk-rocker) walking towards us. Lynne's lips curved into a smile and before too long she was pointing at the poor woman and laughing uncontrollably. Tears were running down her cheeks!

That's what happens with Alzheimer's disease. People lose their filters. The woman walked up and asked Lynne what was so damn funny. I explained what was wrong with

Lynne and she softened visibly. I thought that for a moment Lynne was going to get a hug from a punk rocker. Almost everyone was very kind to Lynne and by extension, to me.

I used to get Lynne ready and dress her before Wendy or Janet arrived, and that was a source of consternation to them. They thought that I should get some rest and let them do it. But I couldn't let go of these jobs. Lynne was evolving from a wife into a daughter to me, and I knew that she enjoyed me looking after her.

Wendy and Janet compensated by doing the laundry and taking Lynne for walks along the lakes near our home. Lynne could not walk far without tiring, so they arranged for a wheelchair so that they could take her on longer walks.

I would always go to the front door to let them in and then bring Lynne downstairs for breakfast before I went to work. Wendy usually had the morning shift, and this little routine had Wendy in stitches!

Lynne would slowly descend the stairs with my help, and then she would stop dead at the stair landing, midway down. She would not move until I gave her a kiss. Wendy would laugh and say to Lynne, "You're looking for a little sugar from Tom, aren't you honey?" And Lynne would giggle quietly and we would finish coming down the stairs.

Janet was usually there when I got home. She was quite talkative and after she got to know me better she would sit in the family room with Lynne and me and fill me in on Lynne's day. She was divorced and she would also talk a bit about her own life and flirt a bit.

Lynne wanted me all to herself, and she would sit there and scowl if Janet stayed too long. Once I guess the flirting crossed the line for Lynne. She looked at Janet sternly and said, "Tom, mine! You go now!" I still smile when I recall the look on Janet's face! My girl still loved me and she was defending her turf!

Another care-giver named Angela came on Wednesdays on Wendy's and Janet's day off. I learned quickly to make certain that the refrigerator was well stocked before she arrived.

Angela decided that Lynne would enjoy sitting in the kitchen and watching while she cooked. Angela was of Portuguese ethnicity and she would raid our fridge and whip up amazing casseroles that would last Lynne and me for about three days.

I reserved Wednesday mornings for Lynne's appointments and booked them well in advance as vacation leave in my electronic calendar. Now and then some mucky-muck would decide that their time was more important than my time with Lynne and book a meeting that conflicted with my time-off. I never blinked. I never missed my time with Lynne.

Some Wednesdays Lynne and I would visit Dr. Campbell. Or go to the dentist or to see Harold for a cut and colour. These were all people who cared about Lynne and truly made a difference in our lives.

Harold lived in an older home and the stairs down to his salon were very steep. Harold would patiently help me get Lynne down the stairs, all the while encouraging Lynne in the best of humour. "Come on, Baby! You can do it!" he would exhort.

I would listen to him tell Lynne jokes and hear her giggle. I am certain that by this time Lynne did not understand half of what Harold was saying, but she enjoyed the inflections in his voice and he made her laugh. Lynne always became agitated when Harold washed her hair, so he would call me in to calm her down and to help him with the wash. By this time it was a two-man job.

Lynne was not yet incontinent, but she did have an accident in Harold's chair once. Harold never batted an eye. He just pretended that it had not happened, and gave me a towel to place under Lynne in the car. He did not want Lynne to feel ashamed. The man was a saint.

Lynne also had gum disease so we went to Dr. Mickflikier's office every couple of months to get Lynne's teeth cleaned and so that the dentist could make sure that I was doing a good job of caring for Lynne's teeth. Lynne had been going there for a long time, and had become close with her dental hygienist (Cheryl) and the receptionist in the office.

When Lynne began to decline, Cheryl asked me to come in and hold Lynne's hand to calm her while Cheryl did her work. Cheryl always talked to Lynne and me about her children and her trips and Lynne would become engrossed in trying to follow the conversation. She would obediently "open wide" when Cheryl requested. Dr. Micflickier was equally patient with Lynne.

Much later, after Lynne had gone into care, I learned that Cheryl worked part-time and that Wednesday was one of her days off. Yet Cheryl would make a special trip downtown on the bus on her day off to look after my Lynne. She never said a word to me about it. She is a kind, gentle woman.

It was because of all of these people, these amazing wonderful people, that I was able to keep Lynne home with me for almost 10 years.

Don't misunderstand me. This was not a cakewalk. There was a period of time where Lynne just wouldn't sleep. The synapses in her brain were firing off at such a random, confusing and rapid rate that she could not lay quiet for more than five minutes.

When Lynne didn't sleep, then neither did I. After five days, I was on my knees. I begged her to stop. I begged her to sleep. Bless her heart. She said, "Trying. Can't help it," as she looked at me with those big brown eyes, full of remorse and concern. It could not have been any better for her than it was for me. In fact, it was probably worse.

I called Dr. Campbell and he prescribed a powerful sedative for Lynne that was supposed to be gradually increased until it became effective. After two more sleepless nights I maxed out the dose, and blessedly, we both slept.

Repetitive behaviour was another problem that Lynne went through that must have been as hard for her as it was for me. Lynne for a period of time would say, "Well I don't know!" She would say it five to ten times a minute for hours. She couldn't help it. Asking her to stop was like asking the rain to stop. She would stop when she was ready. I loved her, but it was exhausting. Eventually that phase of the disease ended.

There was some humour mixed in with the duress. Early in Lynne's decline one Christmas morning Lynne decided that she wanted to go to the Forks for brunch. I said that it was likely closed and she responded, "Of course it's open."

Half way there, Lynne asked me where we were going and I said, "To the Forks for brunch." She looked at me scornfully and said, "What are you thinking? It will be closed!" I then suggested that we go to Salisbury House, which was always open. Lynne never liked Salisbury House and she told me so after I suggested it, but by the time we arrived she had forgotten about her dislike and we had a nice brunch.

There were always new challenges as the disease progressed. It was always changing. And each time Lynne lost some capability to the disease, I mourned the loss of another part of the woman that I loved.

It happened again and again. It was a long, heartbreaking good-bye. Just as I fell in love the new Lynne who had lost another capability she would decline again. I never stopped loving Lynne and because of this, grief became a tangible part of my life.

Urinary incontinence finally became an issue for Lynne. Again, she just couldn't help it. I did many, many loads of sheets in the early morning hours before my Alzheimer's support group clued me in on what to do and acquire: a good, waterproof mattress cover, sheets overlaid with at least one soaker pad and an adult diaper. After that, Lynne was comfortable and dry.

I am not telling you these stories so that you will feel sorry for me. Lynne did her level best and I know that there are many people with Alzheimer's who are far more challenging than Lynne was. None of them can in anyway mitigate the behavioural problems that have beset them. That is my point. These folks need help! Lots of help and understanding. And so do their caregivers.

By this time my son, Dave had moved in with his future wife, Jackie, and I claimed his old bedroom as my own. I missed being in the same bed with Lynne for a number of reasons. I liked to be close to her and I worried that she would try to get out of bed and fall, or wander out and fall down the stairs.

But Lynne and I had a problem. If I rolled over and woke Lynne up, she would not return to sleep and we would both face the next day bone-tired. It happened many times.

I adjusted the door to the master bedroom so that it rubbed against the frame and was hard to open. This was to keep Lynne safe, away from the stairs. For the longest time, the slightest sound would wake me up. I was sleeping with "one eye open," listening for signs of distress in Lynne's room. I was very tired.

Lynne did fall on the stair once. I left her sitting in the kitchen while I went upstairs to get something, and Lynne decided to follow me up the stairs. She got as far as the first landing, and then lost her balance and fell backwards down the stairs. She struck her head on a dining room chair, causing a nasty gash that bled profusely.

I sat Lynne down, comforted her, and then I checked the wound. I got the bleeding to stop, but the wound would need stitches, so off to the hospital emergency room (ER) we went. Unfortunately for us and everyone else in the ER, Winnipeg had experienced an ice-storm that day and the ER was full of slip-and-falls, folks with broken bones. As a result, our wait was very lengthy, about six hours.

Lynne sat quietly waiting, but I noticed her staring intently at a large man in an orange jump suit who was accompanied by two policemen. The man wore handcuffs and leg chains. As the waiting room gradually cleared out, I could hear the conversation taking place between the prisoner and the policemen.

The prisoner was a well-spoken, gentle giant, an ex-soldier who had served in Afghanistan and suffered from post-traumatic stress disorder (PTSD). He had gotten drunk and ended up in a fight that landed him in jail. He asked the military for help for his PTSD while he was in jail. When none was forthcoming, he ran head down into a concrete wall, hoping to be hospitalized so he could get help there.

I felt deeply moved for the man, and at the same time angry and ashamed that our government hadn't helped him. We send these men out to face horrors that can never be erased and they come back broken. Then we don't do nearly enough to fix them.

Eventually, it was Lynne's turn and only the ex-soldier in the orange jump-suit remained. Lynne got her stitches, we went home, I put her to bed and cleaned the blood out of the carpet as I thought about the ex-soldier.

Lynne's only other medical emergency was a seizure that was exactly like an epileptic fit. Lynne always remained in bed while I was getting ready for work in the morning. She seemed content to lie there, and I could keep an eye on her in the bathroom mirror while I shaved.

One morning, I heard a strange choking noise, accompanied by thrashing about. I ran into the bedroom to see Lynne in convulsions in the bed. She was gagging on her tongue, her eyes were rolled back and her body was rigid, with her arms and legs flailing uncontrollably.

I called 911, and while I was talking to the dispatcher, the convulsions stopped and she began to breathe normally. I think that the seizure may have lasted two or three minutes, but it seemed like an eternity to me. Afterwards, Lynne was totally unresponsive. There was not even a glimmer of recognition in her eyes. I was so afraid that I had lost her—that she would not return from where-ever she was.

The first responders arrived in a matter of minutes, while I was still on the telephone talking to the dispatcher. The dispatcher asked whether the front door was locked. I said, "Yes. It is." She said, "You have to leave your wife now and go unlock the door. If you don't, they will knock it down."

I went downstairs and let in the first responders, who turned out to be firefighters trained to deal with medical emergencies. While they were assessing Lynne an ambulance arrived and the medics did a more in-depth examination.

The last thing I remember before they took Lynne to the hospital was this big fireman lifting Lynne like a doll and gently putting her on the gurney. She weighed less than a hundred pounds at that time—not much for someone who was five-foot-six-inches tall.

I was informed by a specialist at the hospital that seizures of this nature were common for people who had Alzheimer's disease. Lynne was given all manner of tests by doctors and technicians that were all very patient and kind.

They prescribed a drug to inhibit the seizures and Lynne was discharged after about thirty-six hours. I was there with her for about thirty of them. I only went home to sleep after I made the nurse promise to call me when she awoke. I didn't want Lynne to come-to in strange surroundings and be afraid.

My return to the workplace was a stark contrast to my private life. In my private life I had many caring individuals that did everything in their power to help me. At work, it was almost the reverse.

When I came back to work my former boss, our director, offered me a senior position in the engineering division. But by the way, you voluntarily relinquished your former position as a division manager and your salary will be downgraded. Your pension will be reduced. We'll let you know who you report to once we figure out how low your salary will be.

I thought about this for about ten seconds before I sought legal counsel. I was fortunate on two fronts. After I was hospitalized, I was still on the email circulation list for the management team. I had received an email that clearly contradicted the notion that I had voluntarily relinquished my old position. I don't think that I was intended to receive it. I printed it and I saved an electronic copy of the file.

In addition, the city solicitor had just retired. Marvin Samphir and I were not close friends, but we knew one another fairly well and he knew an injustice when he saw one. So Marvin agreed to review correspondence and to provide advice as to how to respond.

He knew our system well. We both agreed that it would best if he worked in the background, in order to avoid escalating the issue. And so we negotiated back and forth. I would receive a letter from the city and then I would pen a response. Marvin would review it and tone it down when my emotions surfaced. He would provide advice on matters of labour law.

The final letter upon which the terms of my employment where based saved me from many pitfalls during my remaining years with the city, and Marvin earned every dime of his fee. My salary and by extension my pension were protected. In five years I could retire and spend more time with Lynne. Most importantly, I could afford to pay for her care once she moved into a personal care home. This would be a considerable cost.

I returned to work as the project director for the Water Treatment Program. This was a high profile position responsible for the design and construction of Winnipeg's first water treatment plant, a facility which cost over two hundred and eighty million dollars to construct.

There were staff in the Engineering Division that coveted that position and they did not welcome me back. From my point of view, not enough was done to counteract that resistance at a management level. I was left off circulation lists. I was not invited to team meetings. I was not welcome.

At the same time, the woman that I had mentored when she reported to me, and that I had recommended for my position when I underwent surgery seemed intent upon making my work as difficult as possible.

What the hell! I did what I have always done. I got the damn job done. But I wondered how people who knew me and worked with me could do these things that were so hurtful and detracted from my only reason for living at that time—taking care of my wife. They are not on my Christmas card list.

After much pressuring from folks in my Caregivers support group (and my son and my doctor and my friends), I finally had Lynne paneled and placed on a waiting list for a personal care home (PCH). The recurring theme seemed to be, "You are burning out and placing your health in jeopardy. You won't do Lynne any good if you are in the hospital or dead!"

There was some truth to what they were saying. Many caregivers suffer mental or physical breakdowns due to the stress and the unending work of providing care to a loved one. I remembered the words of the ER nurse when I told her that I was going to look after Lynne. "Don't die trying."

I toured about six PCHs. I winnowed the list down to two and finally one choice. I was very thorough. I knew that this was going to be Lynne's last home and I wanted to make the best possible choice for Lynne. And I think I did.

The decision to place Lynne in care resulted in a need for me to relocate, which I will talk about in a little while. First I'd like to tell you about my last two wonderful memories of our home...

The first was Lynne's sixtieth birthday party. There were just David, Jackie, Lynne and me in attendance. It was a gala event for Lynne! We had the perquisite Jeanne's cake with candles and ice cream. When we sang *Happy Birthday* and urged Lynne to blow out the candles, she sat there, grinning from ear to ear until I helped her blow them out. Then she scarfed down two pieces of cake with ice cream!

The second was Dave and Jackie's wedding. Dave and Jackie were married outdoors at a restaurant called Terrace Fifty-Five in Assiniboine Park. It is a beautiful setting and as you will learn later, the venue became something of a family tradition.

We held the wedding reception at the restaurant. Lynne could not attend the wedding. It would have been too hard on her. So the kids decided to have the cake-cutting ceremony at our home so Lynne could participate.

Lynne's brother Jack was able to attend as well. I don't think Lynne remembered Jack when she first saw him, but she smiled when she heard his voice and I knew then that she remembered him (people with Alzheimer's tend to remember voices long after they forget faces). I have a photograph of Lynne sitting quietly with Jack's arm around her, smiling her "Mona Lisa" smile.

Lynne's face lit up when she saw Dave and Jackie arrive in their wedding garb and she said, "Pretty!" She seemed mesmerized by Jackie's wedding dress, and for weeks after she became excited every time she saw a wedding gown on TV.

Sadly, by then Lynne's sun was setting quickly and it was becoming beyond my capacity to provide the care that she needed. Lynne would soon be going to live at Lion's Personal Care home, but first she would spend a short time in another new home.

We move one last time

Once I decided that Lion's was the best PCH for Lynne, the notion of moving just kind of crept into my mind. I needed to be close to Lynne, and I didn't want to be knocking around our old home, full of ghosts.

I started to consider alternatives when I had the time. I needed to be close to downtown and I didn't want the work of an old house (I would be busy visiting Lynne), so I thought I would likely end up in a condo.

The problem I had was that I had acquired an old British sports car and I was attached to the darn thing. A condo doesn't work well if you have a British car in one of your parking spaces, in need of repair!

As I was driving home one day, I saw an open house sign on Osborne, just south of downtown. I followed the signs and came to a brand new architecturally designed in-fill home on Walker Avenue, close to downtown. It was very nice, but it was too large for my needs and it lacked a garage.

I spoke to the agent and told him that the house was gorgeous, but wouldn't work for me. He said that the architect had another open house the same day on the other side of Osborne, down by the river, and that I should have a look at it—it might be more to my liking.

I went over and checked it out. It was a stunning modern home, but too large, with a garage that was too small. I told the agent how impressed I was with the house, and he said, "Would you like to meet the architect? He's right over there."

That's how I met Will Richard. Will is a crusty architect with great talent, a love for in-fill housing and a generous heart.

When I told Will how much I liked the home his first words were, "Then why don't you buy it?" I explained what didn't work for me in the house and then I told him that I really wanted to wait a year, until my wife was in care. Will asked me why my wife was going into care and I gave him the abbreviated version of our sad story.

He was quiet for a moment. Then he said, "What did you think of the house on Walker?" I said I liked it, but I would prefer a better level of finish. Will said that the fellow that had the Walker property for sale (Steven) also owned an in-fill lot down the street, across from the park. He said that he would be happy to introduce us and if we could make a deal Will would do some preliminary plans for budget purposes at no cost.

Steven's property never went on the market. He and I hit it off and I bought the property. Will designed a home exactly to my needs and after three months of zoning tribulations (it was too modern for some of my neighbours' tastes) and five months of construction I had my new house, close to where my Lynne would be living.

A five month construction period for a custom build is very fast. Many of the trades working on the house knew about Lynne, and I know that they went "above and beyond." Albert framed our home and did the finish carpentry. After he was finished (he did a fine job) he stopped by a couple of times to help me with jobs he knew I couldn't do on my own.

Phil (our electrician and a personal friend), worked like a demon to have the wiring complete in time for the insulation, vapour barrier and drywall. Will designed and built a beautiful solid maple stair for the house, with as he put it, "a nice gentle step" for Lynne and a large walk-in shower was installed off the master suite to bathe Lynne, if she hadn't been admitted by the time I had to move.

Will's buddy Kel helped install the stair. Will even took me to Kel's home to show me the style of sink he was planning for my kitchen. When I paid Will his fee for his work, I told him it seemed low. Will simply said gruffly, "I like you."

Once again, the Universe had conspired to help Lynne and me along towards the end of our story. There was another connection with Will and Kel that became very important to me, but you will hear about that later in the book.

The social worker that was working on Lynne's admission at Lion's was named Judy. She knew the moment that we met that I was having a terrible time letting go of Lynne. She very graciously said, "You're on our list now, but I have some latitude and Lynne has some special placement requirements. You call me when you are six months from being ready to let her go and I will begin the process."

So I finally made the call, even though in my heart of hearts, I wasn't ready. I am not sure that you are ever ready. Then time dragged on. Judy had a specific wing on a specific floor in mind for Lynne. Lynne needed a nice, quiet environment like she had at home. And the only time that there are vacancies is... you guessed it—when someone dies. And that is hard to predict. Consequently, despite my best planning and efforts we had to sell our family home and move before Lynne went into care.

When I look back at that time, it's all a blur to me— having the new house built, marketing our old home and moving while caring for Lynne exhausted me. I know that it was difficult for Lynne as well. Nevertheless there was a little bit of humour mixed in with all the work and change.

We needed to have an open-house as part of our realtor's marketing plan, and that meant that Lynne and I had to be out of the house for several hours. The problem was—what would we do? We couldn't go for a walk because Lynne couldn't walk very far without getting tired. We could sit somewhere for a while, or we could drive around a bit (Lynne was always soothed by drives), or maybe we could go for a meal.

Other than going to our favourite spot at the Forks for breakfast Lynne and I hadn't been to a restaurant for a long while. There were several reasons for this. Lynne enjoyed the familiar dishes that I prepared for her. And as her capabilities declined, she became embarrassed that she couldn't order on her own. And finally, she could no longer handle cutlery and I had to feed her while eating my own meal. But today we were going out for dinner! We had time to kill and it was time to eat.

We went to a restaurant at the Forks. There was disabled parking nearby, so Lynne didn't need to walk too far, and I thought that the familiar surroundings would soothe her. I helped Lynne into the restaurant and got her seated in a quiet area. The waitress brought our menus and I read the selections that I thought Lynne would enjoy out-loud to her.

I am certain that she didn't understand most of what I said, but it was important to me that she felt as though the menu choice was hers. We settled on salmon with mango sauce for Lynne. I ordered for both of us and the waitress repeated Lynne's order to her and said, "Have I got that right?" Lynne said, "OK!" in a happy voice. Then off the waitress went.

The funny part was the look on the waitress's face when she brought our orders. The mango sauce on Lynne's salmon was a bright orange and Lynne took one look at it and said very loudly, "Eeeww!" I thought that the waitress was going to have a fit! I then realized that I should have explained a little about Lynne when we sat down.

I told the waitress not to worry. Lynne had Alzheimer's disease and she was just reacting to the colour of the sauce, but everything would be fine. I then asked Lynne to try a little taste of it and she loudly proclaimed, "Mmm!" I fed her everything on her plate and then shared a dessert with her before we left. The surrounding diners and the waitress were very kind. I tipped big.

The house was sold fairly quickly and it was time to move. There is an image from the day we moved that is etched forever in my memory. I had asked my son Dave to make a deal with some buddies to help out. We weren't moving far, and that way things could be moved in a logical sequence and placed where I needed them in the new house.

There was some furniture and other stuff that either wouldn't fit in the new house or that I didn't want, and Dave and Jackie got first call on this, followed by Dave's helpers. The whole thing was fairly efficient. I rented a large truck. The young guys did the heavy lifting and I drove the truck and directed traffic. One of Lynne's regular caregivers from homecare came to be with Lynne while all this was going on.

With all the hub-bub, I never thought about the effect this would have on Lynne. I had made a terrible mistake. I should have brought her over to the new house before the old one was empty. At the end of the day, there was Lynne, sitting forlornly on a kitchen chair, next to her caregiver in an empty house, a house that Lynne had lived in for twenty-one years.

I felt physically ill when I saw Lynne sitting there, sadly wondering what had happened. I hugged her and took her to our new home. She was comforted by the sight of the old familiar furniture. I stayed very close to Lynne for the rest of the day. She needed me.

Lynne's brief stay in our new home in Riverview was difficult for both of us. Both Janet and Wendy wanted to care for Lynne until she moved to Lion's, but the mucky-mucks at Homecare wouldn't allow them to work out of their assigned area. This meant that Lynne had to adapt to a whole new staff and I had to orient them as to Lynne's needs and our routines.

To make matters even worse, the management in the new catchment area where we lived failed to set up a proper schedule for caregivers. Sometimes, they didn't show up and I couldn't go to work. Sometimes, they were late. Sometimes, I would go to work after orienting a new worker and come home to find a totally different person in the house—someone who hadn't even been told that Lynne had Alzheimer's disease! Sometimes Lynne had soiled herself.

"Oh, she needs help with the toileting? Nobody told me that!" Really? *Do you have a sense of smell?*

I went ballistic and went up the food chain right to the Minister of Health's office. After that things improved, but I couldn't help, but think about some of the elderly folks in my Caregivers Support Group. Would they have been able to raise hell in this situation and have it corrected? Or would all the trouble have broken them?

So I began to request formal, written responses to the issues I had raised. I wasn't interested in apologies. I wanted solutions. I am proud to say that, at least in a very small way, I was able to change some of Homecare's policies to better support their clients.

Lions

After about two months in our new home with Lynne I received a call from Judy. They had a suitable spot for Lynne. She could come the next day. I said that I would like a bit of time to prepare Lynne and myself for this change.

Judy said that she understood, but effective the next day, I would have to start paying for the cost of care at Lion's. I said that, after all that time, a little bit of money didn't matter.

Everyone in my support group had told me, "Don't go alone when you take Lynne to Lion's. It will be very, very hard for you." So I called Dave and asked if he and Jackie could come with me in a couple of days when I took Mom to Lion's. They agreed, although I am certain that it was almost as difficult for them as for me.

I moved most of Lynne's things over ahead of time, along with a TV and a familiar chair. Then we took Lynne to Lion's. Lynne's cognitive abilities had declined significantly by then, but when she got off the elevator and saw all the elderly women sitting by the nurses' station she said, "Not me!" She knew what was happening. We stayed with Lynne for about an hour and the staff came and introduced themselves to Lynne and to us, and then we went home.

Lynne was sixty years old then. She was the youngest resident at Lion's.

I made Dave and Jackie dinner and we talked a little about Lynne. They both said not to worry, that everything would be fine. I had done everything that I could. Lynne's brother, Jack, called and told me the same thing. He said he couldn't have asked for a better husband for his sister. At this point I was doing OK.

David and Jackie went home and I thought *I need to go back and see how Lynne is doing.* When I went back to Lion's, Lynne was sitting in her room alone. The staff had left the TV on for her and they popped in now and then to check on her.

Lynne was happy to see me and I sat on the arm of her chair and snuggled her a bit, for another hour or so. She got drowsy and the staff put her to bed and I went home to my empty house. I had a couple of glasses of wine and I cried until I thought I had nothing left in me. Then I finished the bottle and cried some more, until I fell asleep.

I felt enormous guilt when I placed Lynne in care. My mind told me that I had done the right thing. I could no longer provide the care that she needed, and I was exhausted. The recent problems with Homecare only exacerbated the situation. Lynne needed consistent care by trained, compassionate professionals. But my heart told me that I had betrayed Lynne. I had let her down. The guilt tore at my insides.

Although the transition was very difficult for both Lynne and me, Lion's turned out to be the best thing that could have happened to both of us. Initially Lynne and I missed each other terribly, but I visited Lynne every day after work, and we both adjusted.

Lynne usually had a smile for me when I arrived. I fed her dinner, took her for a walk around the floor and then watched a little TV with her. On weekends I went at lunchtime. Lynne settled in and received the care that she needed, and the staff there treated both of us like family. I can't thank them enough for all that they did for Lynne and me.

My new best friend...

I used to get together with a good friend of mine named Jim for a few beers and a dinner once a month, both before and after Lynne went into care. Actually, we continue to carry out that ritual to this very day.

Jim's father passed away after suffering with Alzheimer's disease, so Jim had a pretty good idea of what I was going through. He gave me a lot of moral support and advice about how to cope. He also helped me deal with the guilt that overcame me when I placed Lynne in care. Jim always had good advice and I listened carefully to what he had to say.

After Lynne went into care, Jim asked me when I had last taken a vacation. I thought about it and realized that it had been about five years. Five years is a long time when you are working full-time and caring for a loved one with Alzheimer's disease.

I actually could have taken a week here or there while Lynne was still at home, but I would have had to place her into short term care and I just couldn't do it. It would have been too difficult for Lynne. She would have been lonely and frightened and I would have been miserable the whole time that she was away.

Jim, after a couple of beers, in his usually forthright manner, said, "Tommy, you look like crap! Why don't you take a week off and go someplace warm!" It was November and in Winnipeg, winter was already upon us.

I thought about it. Lynne seemed to be adapting well to her new environment and I didn't think it would be too hard on her if I was away for a week. I decided to fly to Palm Springs and spend a week in our time-share in Indian Wells. It was a week that changed my life, in a couple of ways.

My time in Indian Wells was bittersweet. A melange of memories of Lynne and me at the time-share came flooding back. They were all good memories, but I missed Lynne (both Lynnes actually—the one with Alzheimer's disease and the old Lynne, before Alzheimer's) terribly.

Let me explain. While I was caring for Lynne, I had never allowed myself to remember her when she was healthy. I think that this was a protective mechanism on my part. The grief would have likely crippled me. So there I was at the time-share, remembering all the good times we had there when Lynne was healthy while calling Lion's every other day to make sure that Lynne (with Alzheimer's) was OK.

I spent my days running in the morning and then sitting on the patio drinking coffee and reading the local paper. In the evening, I would barbeque a dinner and have a couple of glasses of wine, also on the patio. My patio was next to a sidewalk that led to the parking area and other residents would say hello and chat now and then.

And that's how I met Mary Sue. At the time, Mary Sue lived across the way from me and she was coming and going a lot. She was a representative for a clothing manufacturer and the coming and going usually involved the transport of one or more large boxes.

On this particular morning, I was sipping coffee and watching bemusedly as this perky little thing carried one box in her arms and kicked another along the sidewalk towards her car. There was a dog (Abbey, I later learned) involved in this production as well. I asked her if she we would like some help and she declined. I thought *She probably thinks I am about to hit on her. Oh well...* and I went back to my paper.

I looked up and realized that Mary Sue was standing next to my patio. She introduced herself and her dog Abbey and after a bit of back and forth, off to work she went.

There was a full moon while I was in Indian Wells and I recalled how much Lynne loved the moon. We would walk along the base of the Santa Rosa Mountains and gaze up at the stars and the moon. The sky was so clear that the stars seemed to carpet the sky. So I would walk under that moon and grieve for the Lynne that I once knew...

The second time that I ran into Mary Sue was after I had gone for a walk under that full moon and I was thinking about Lynne. I came walking up behind her out of the dark and said, "Hello." She didn't hear me coming and she jumped about a foot!

We spoke briefly and Mary Sue looked at me curiously and asked me if I would like to come in for a glass of wine. I agreed. We had a glass of wine and Mary Sue began to gently prod. She had seen the look on my face and she wanted to know the story behind it. I hadn't realized that my grief was so transparent. Mary Sue is a very good listener and it wasn't long before I had told her all about Lynne and me.

I must have been looking into space as I told my story, and when I looked up at Mary Sue she was staring at me with tears in her eyes. Mary Sue believes firmly in God's power and she said, "I will say a prayer for both of you."

Then she told me her story. She was estranged from her partner, Rob, but they were trying to sort things out. She told me what was wrong with their relationship and said that she wished that Rob loved her even half as much as I obviously loved Lynne.

She said that I should be very proud of the way that I had been there for Lynne, through thick and thin. I simply said that you can go through a lot for the right reason, and that for me the reason was love. And that is how I met my new best friend, Mary Sue. We were two lonely people who began the evening as strangers and ended up baring our souls to each other.

After that we corresponded by email often, sharing our problems and offering advice to one another. We would speak on the phone now and then, but for some reason email seemed to work best for us.

I would update Mary Sue on Lynne's ups and downs and because of this I have what amounts to a weekly journal of Lynne's life at Lion's until her passing. Mary Sue was so moved by it that she urged me to write this book, to give others in a similar situation some hope. We always visit whenever I am in Indian Wells, and we often reminisce about Lynne.

Mary Sue moved back with Rob, for a while, but that didn't work out and I was glad of it. It was my firm belief that Mary Sue deserved happiness and Rob couldn't deliver. After that, I would regard each new relationship that Mary Sue became involved in with the scrutiny of an overly-protective brother.

Mary Sue and I never became romantically involved, although I think that at some time or other we both thought about it. I know that I did. But we never thought about it at the *same* time and it is just as well.

Long distance relationships don't often work out and at least for me, our friendship was something I did not want to jeopardize. I once told her that she was not a lover, but she was certainly someone that I loved. Our friendship still endures. There is only one woman alive that I am closer to than Mary Sue and you will meet her very soon.

Mary Sue became a safe-harbour for me. I could share all the trials I experienced in dealing with Lynne's decline without fear of embarrassment or criticism. For a period of time she was truly a life-saver.

The other change that Mary Sue precipitated in my life was a realization of just how lonely I had become. This provided the impetus to begin dating again, and I'll tell you about those experiences in a while. I received lots of good advice from Mary Sue about the experiences covered there.

But first, I need to tell you what happened when I returned to Winnipeg, after my vacation in Indian Wells.

Back to reality

I returned to Winnipeg from Indian Wells in during the first week of December, 2008. I went to visit with Lynne twice that day, and I didn't think she knew me anymore. She wouldn't smile for me anymore. No smiles. She had a small seizure while I was there, and she seemed comforted when I held her, and kissed her forehead, but I didn't think that she knew me.

Lord, forgive me and help me. I felt that I was responsible for Lynne's condition, that if I had stayed in Winnipeg instead of going away, maybe she would have been OK. I cried all that evening, and I couldn't seem to make it stop. The guilt overwhelmed me.

I visited Lynne each day after work. Usually, our routine entailed me feeding her dinner while telling her about my day and trying to make her laugh, or at least smile. Some days, I came at noon as well. I would always take her for a walk around the floor and spend some time watching TV with her after dinner. Gradually, we seemed to reconnect, until one Friday, everything (at least to me) seemed wonderful again!

I wrote this note to Mary Sue, who was quite worried about Lynne and me: *When I stopped to visit with Lynne on Friday after work, she was having a great day! She talked a little, and I got a couple of smiles from her!*

Mary Sue, when I left I was walking on air! Of course, by Saturday that was all gone. Ups and downs. They are very hard, but that is the essence of the disease. Sometimes I think I just need to toughen up a bit, but I don't want to lose what I feel for Lynne.

Mary Sue wrote these words of encouragement. "You've been the best husband anyone could ask for—even if you had bad days—they were nothing compared to what most people go through. Allow yourself to be proud of what you have done with Lynne—I know she is amazed at your loyalty, compassion and the love you have shown her."

My first day back with Lynne was very difficult and painful. Mary Sue's words of encouragement helped me a great deal.

Of course, life outside of Lion's went on as well, but it almost seemed to be in a parallel universe.

I went out with my buddy Jim on a Wednesday night. He and his wife Chris were going to Florida for a month in early January, and this was our last hurrah before the trip. Jim and I go back about thirty years. He looks and acts like someone named "Bubba" from the south, but he is a very bright guy.

We had a really good time, and consequently I worked out of my home office on Thursday morning. Jim was working on me. He kept saying, "You don't need the money, retire now and play with your cars and take up golf!" I kept saying, "I do need the money, and I also need something to fill in my days until I get a life!" It's amazing how much beer you can drink while you have these deep discussions!

A fellow engineer named Chris Macey lost his wife to cancer about that time. I was able to attend Darlene's (Chris's wife) funeral on a Thursday. I wasn't certain right up to the end whether I would be able to do it, but I did. I didn't know Darlene very well, but I knew Chris for twenty-five years.

He is a brilliant engineer, a real renaissance man. He put together a computerized slide show of Darlene's life, complete with period music of their life together, and at the end of it all I thought I knew her well, or at least I knew Darlene as Chris saw her. Chris seemed genuinely pleased to see me, so I was glad I went.

There were about three hundred folks in attendance. Winnipeg is a small town in a professional sense, and I saw a lot of people that I'd lost touch with during Lynne's illness. I didn't stay long; it was too hard for me to answer the well-intended questions about Lynne. The whole thing made we wonder how I would ever survive Lynne's passing, when the time finally came.

I went to visit Lynne a couple of times on December 24th, and spent Christmas eve wrapping gifts and sipping wine (a little too much, from the feel of my head the next day!). It was a little lonely, but not too bad. It was my first Christmas in thirty one years that Lynne and I were not under the same roof.

On Christmas day I visited Lynne at lunch. I fed her and then opened her gifts for her. I used to make it my mission to find her something truly extravagant, that I knew she would enjoy, but never buy for herself. This year I couldn't do that—the laundry at the care home was pretty rough on clothes, so it needed to be "wash and wear."

I got her a track suit and a couple of tops, socks etc. Things she needed. I think that she enjoyed it more when I was unwrapping the presents for her, than when she saw the gifts. The one exception was a box of Laura Secord chocolates. Women and chocolates! After I opened the box and put one in Lynne's mouth, her eyes kind of widened and she said, "Oh!" in the cutest way! It put a smile on my face.

My son Dave and his wife Jackie came over in the afternoon and we exchanged gifts and had Christmas dinner. My sister and Lynne's brother Jack both called, as well as my friend Jim. I think that Jim was checking up on me. He called in the morning and wanted to know if the tree was up and dinner was under control!

Through the efforts of many good friends, I was getting the guilt thing under control and surviving the Christmas season. Jack made a point of thanking me (again) for all I had done for Lynne, and said that from where he sat, I had done more than anyone could reasonably expect or even hope for! Those words meant a lot to me.

We have a tradition in our house. If I can stay awake until midnight on New Year's Eve, I open the front door of our home to let the old year out and the New Year in, and toast them both—*Good times gone by and good times to come!* Lynne and I did that for as long as I can remember.

That year I did it alone, and it didn't seem too bad. But it did take a few glasses of wine and a stiff Scotch to get there. I watched the New Year's Eve fireworks at the Forks from our front patio door and went to bed.

During that period, I was slowly putting the finishing touches of my house, as well as holding down a fairly demanding job, but my main focus remained getting the most out of my visits with Lynne and staying connected.

Lynne finally adjusted to her new surroundings and seemed more content. I visited with her on most days on the way home from work, but I was finally able to miss a day (no more guilt!), when I had another commitment. She would often smile and say, "Oh!" when I arrived. I was even able to get a giggle from her now and then. In our own way, we were able to enjoy our time together. I gave that a bit of thought. Most people with Alzheimer's disease are placed in care within three to five years after diagnosis. I was able to keep Lynne at home for almost ten years, and I know that I truly made a difference for her.

I finally allowed myself to feel proud of what I had done! Lynne's illness tested me in ways that I could not have imagined, and it made me a better person than I ever thought that I could be. I think that I finally understood what is important in life. Lynne's care was fundamentally a labour of love, and it was more important to me than anything else I had ever done. It was very hard, but it fulfilled me. *Better late than never.*

"Extra-Miler" was a term that Lynne introduced me to. It is someone who has the stamina and the courage to go the distance and then some. Lynne was an extra-miler, and she knew one when she saw one. She told me that I was an extra-miler soon after I met her, and that made me proud. History had proven her right.

But even though I had managed to deal with my guilt, grief still held me in an iron grip. They call Alzheimer's disease "the long good-bye." You lose your loved one a bit at a time. Then you grow to love the "new" person, and you lose part of them. And so it goes, on and on. Each time, the pain brings you to your knees.

Lynne was now at the stage where her mental capacity was sadly very similar to that of a very young child. She was very proud when I took her by the hands and led her down the hall for a walk, and told her what a good girl she was. It made her smile.

She had to try very hard to take that walk, and she deserved to be proud. She couldn't master speech anymore, so she made her feelings known through sounds. She liked to be held and snuggled. And it broke my heart, over and over again, when I lost any part of what she had now become.

When I stopped to visit Lynne one evening in late January, she didn't seem herself. I fed her dinner, and then took her for the ritual walk to the lounge, to show her the city lights, and then for our usual walk around the floor. I did that to try to preserve her ability to walk, so that she won't be restricted to a wheel chair too soon.

About half way around the floor, she stiffened and tilted her head back, with her eyes rolled back as well. I called to Ted (one of the orderlies) to quickly bring a chair. Even though she only weighed about 100 pounds, it was all I could do to keep her from falling and hurting herself.

We got her into the chair, and I wheeled her back to her room, and lifted her into her arm chair. She was so afraid! I hugged her and patted her to calm her down, and it helped, but she was terrified! It was heart wrenching to see her like that.

Yet the next day when I visited, Lynne was just fine. They had given her a bath just before dinner, and she was cosy and warm in her nightgown and housecoat, and happy as a clam. The previous evening I was devastated. The next day I was holding my own. But it reminded me how difficult the future might be. I needed to take the easy road, and not subject myself to unnecessary pressures.

I decided to take the next week off and just "shut down." I would work on my Triumph sports car, visit Lynne and catch up on a few things. The incident with Lynne wore me out. Next week was our thirtieth anniversary, and I knew it would make me sad. Life can be tough on us extra-milers!

It was time for a sip of single malt scotch and bed.

Dating, Cancer and Commitment

Talking to Mary Sue while I was in Indian Wells made me realize just how lonely I had become. I told her about this and she urged me to "get out there"—to go on a few dates.

I wasn't certain that I was ready to do this. I visited Lynne every day and I was certain that I would feel guilty about dating. Mary Sue pretty much said, "You will feel whatever your conscience lets you feel, but you and I both know that Lynne would not want you to be alone. She would want you to be happy."

My sister (never shy or short of words) had a more direct message, and I quote: "You've done way more than you should have. I thought you were going to give yourself a heart attack! It's time for you to start living your life and find yourself a nice girl, or you're going to end up a lonely old man!"

However, there were some problems with this. Lynne was still my wife and I wasn't certain that I was prepared to see other women while she was still alive. I was also vulnerable—I honestly didn't think I would ever stop grieving for Lynne even after she was gone.

I hoped that sooner or later, I would be able to manage the grief, and perhaps encounter someone who could bring some light into my life. But scars take time to heal, and if you rush things you can get hurt. I began to wrestle with the notion of dating. It took me quite a while to get through this process.

What qualities were important to me in a woman? For me, the categories were friend, partner and lover. Interestingly, one doesn't necessarily follow the other.

Friends are not always lovers. Lovers are not always friends. It was the same for partners. I wanted it all. I wanted someone that I could enjoy spending time with (friend), who I could collaborate with to resolve life's problems (partner), and someone that made my heart beat a little faster every time I looked at them (lover).

Although my life was a train wreck at that point in time, I'd had the good fortune to have all three of those qualities in Lynne for about twenty-five of my last thirty years. I had no intention of settling for less at this late stage of my life. Although I thought I might end up writing a play called, *A Good Woman is Hard to Find!* in my retirement.

I finally decided that it was worth the risk, but that I needed to be totally up front about my personal situation and the fact that Lynne was my first priority. If I didn't enjoy dating or found it too difficult, I would just stop. It is with that background that a man whose last date occurred before the Internet had been invented was introduced to the world of Internet dating. As I discovered, it is not for the faint of heart...

When I went online, the first thing I learned was that there were a lot of women out there who wanted to meet a fifty-something guy with an ailing wife. They came in all shapes and sizes.

I also learned that their profiles and photos sometimes had only the slightest connection to reality. Let's just say there were some surprises! But I did meet some genuinely nice, interesting women, and as you will learn, one of them turned out to be a "keeper!" Luckily for me, she felt the same way.

Here are some of my "dating" stories:

First Date: Dulcie is the first woman I dated, after thirty years of marriage! She's a smart, personable lady and we hit it off famously, but there were no "sparks" on my end, or hers either. We remained friends, and she found her perfect man subsequently. Dulcie emailed one day out of the blue and asked me if I'd go for lunch with her. So I did.

It turned out that Dulcie had decided that one of her close friends and I would be perfect together, and she was on a mission to make that happen. But first, I had to answer a series of skill testing questions to ensure compatibility over lunch. And of course, agree to see her friend.

I had a few questions of my own. She told me about her friend, Estelle. I said, "What the heck, set it up! Just don't be angry with either of us if it doesn't work out." After that, Dulcie bought me lunch and we stopped off to shop for a couple of items (lamps for my living room, to go with my new tables, and an accent piece) for my house. We were like an old married couple when we got together!

Then she took me to her condo to provide recommendations on how to fix her shower and to have a scotch with her new love, Darrel. It was a pleasant if somewhat bizarre day. Estelle and I didn't work out, mainly because, about the time that I met her, I met another woman who turned out to be the second love of my life.

Irony: One evening, after I visited with Lynne, I had a date for drinks with a lady named Jane. Jane was quite pretty, but based on my experience, it was indeed only "skin deep."

We were to meet at seven-thirty p.m. at a bar, and I was late. It had taken me a little longer than normal to feed Lynne her dinner. When I finally arrived, Jane was already nursing a drink. After I sat down, she proceeded to tell me that if our relationship was ever to flourish, I needed to "let go" of Lynne and stop going to visit every day. Jane needed to come first.

I did something that I had never done before. I said excuse me, I'll be back in a moment. Then I went to the back of the bar and settled the bill. I went back to the table and informed Jane that Lynne had more courage and grace than anyone I had ever met—more than Jane would ever possess and I would *never* abandon her.

Jane said, "Well, you don't know what you're missing!" I said I was pretty sure I knew exactly what I was missing and I walked out the door.

Inquisitive Children: One weekend, my son Dave and his wife Jackie were over for dinner. They were very curious about who I was dating and not too shy about asking! It was a bit of an inquisition. I told them that by that time I was seeing two women, Anita and Deborah.

Jackie began to grill me about Anita. First of all, *did I like her a lot?* I said *no*, that we had been out a few times, and although the first time was OK, I sensed something I didn't care for on subsequent dates. I didn't say what.

Jackie continued to cross examine me about details. What did the woman look like? Where does she live, and finally, what is her last name? I coughed up the information, and then she blurted out, "That's my best friend's Dad's ex! She's an evil, mean woman and she took him for everything she could! You stay away from her!"

I was touched by how protective she was of me. And ironically, that was why I had decided not to see Anita again. She seemed too interested in my assets.

Airport Pick-up: Deborah and I connected through a site called Chemistry.com. The site conducted a very comprehensive personality profile and matched you with compatible personalities. Their assessment indicated that Deborah and I were about a ninety-five percent match. In hindsight, they had us nailed.

We first met at the airport in Winnipeg when Deborah picked me up on my way back from Indian Wells. We had already spoken on the telephone a few time and we both knew that we had a common acquaintance named Will Richard. Will was the architect that had designed my new home and he used to live down the street from Deborah and her ex. That's why Deborah was comfortable coming to the airport to drive me home on a first date.

Our first meeting was somewhat traumatic for me. I cleared customs and scanned the waiting area for someone that resembled Deborah's on-line photo. By this time I knew that these photographs often only bore a passing resemblance to the woman, so close counted.

I walked up to a likely candidate and asked, "Excuse me, are you Deborah?" The woman looked me up and down and then said quite loudly, "No, but nice try!" Then she called out in a very loud voice to the rest of the people in the room, "Anyone here named Deborah?" I slinked out the waiting room as quickly as possible to text Deborah and find out where she was.

It turned out that Deborah was running late and was just pulling into the loading zone. When I told her what happened she thought it was pretty funny! Me, not so much.

In addition to providing me with a ride home from the airport, Deborah turned up with some cheese and fruit, a bottle of red wine and some fresh milk (I had been away for a week). Dating had sure changed since I was young.

What Deborah didn't know was that I had already met Deborah's ex, Kel. Kel had helped Will construct a custom stair for my home and I had been over to Kel's house (Deborah's old house) to check out the butterfly sink configuration in his kitchen.

When Deborah and I arrived home from the airport, I took her on a tour of the house. When she saw my kitchen she said, "I used to have a sink just like that." I said, "I know. I've seen it." Then I told her about my connection to Kel and we had a good laugh. We truly live in a small world.

In many ways, Deborah was a perfect match for me. She had a Master's Degree in social work and worked as professional lead in a hospital, so she understood the challenges that I had with Lynne. She also had a private practice, providing counselling to individuals and couples and Lord knows I needed a bit of that!

I learned early on that when she interjected, "Tell me more about that" into one of our conversations, I should consider my response carefully. It wasn't long before

Deborah and I were seeing a lot of one another. She hadn't asked, but I sensed she would like an exclusive relationship.

I wasn't there yet. I needed to have all the boxes ticked—friend, partner and lover. But with Deborah, there were plenty of sparks and a lot of laughter, so I wanted to see how the other categories developed.

Fun: Deborah and I went for breakfast to a falafel place on Corydon Ave. It's a pretty trendy area, about five minutes from where I live. If you have ever watched *Seinfeld* you have likely seen a character called "the soup Nazi." The owner of the restaurant reminded me of him.

Deborah and the owner's wife were friends, so when we showed up, even though the place was beyond full, he said, "I'll kick somebody out!" and proceeded to roam the restaurant looking for people that were lingering over coffee, and telling them to go pay their bill.

Apparently, he did this all the time, and did not discriminate. It didn't matter whether you were a "regular," a friend or a minor celebrity (there were a few in the crowd) out you went. It was kind of fun, and the food was incredible. The owner was from Israel, and the fusion of his culture and North American breakfast fare was great.

Second Thoughts: One night while I was on my own, I thought a little about my dating experiences. I had told Annette (the gold digger), "no thanks." If I ever saw Jane again, she would likely try to run me over with her car—and Estelle, although she was a very nice person, was not for me.

Deborah hadn't affected me the way that Lynne had when we met. She wasn't a bolt out of the sky. She was more of a slow fire. Yet, she was slowly winning me over, and I found myself growing more and more fond of her. Deborah was a good person and she understood my love for Lynne.

Good Times: Deborah took me to a Diana Krall concert one week—good jazz and some old standards. Diana Krall was on piano, backed up by a trio (guitar, drums and bass) and the Winnipeg Symphony orchestra. It was a great show. It had been a while since I was able to take in shows, and it was nice.

I missed Lynne horribly when I went. She really enjoyed that type of thing. But Deborah seemed to understand. I began to think that as long as Deborah gave me my space, things could work out with us. By that time, I had dated quite a few women, but in all honesty, none as good-hearted as Deborah.

Mary Sue had been privy to all these goings-on through email, and she pushed me a little on Deborah and my relationship. Why had I not yet been able to commit to Deborah? Was it because I couldn't love another woman while Lynne was still in my heart? It was food for thought. I had two kinds of love for Lynne. That much I knew.

I loved the memory of the woman whom I had married, but that woman was gone. Yet I loved the woman Lynne had become. That love was more like the love that a parent feels for a child than what a man feels for his wife. It wasn't a barrier to loving a new partner.

So where did that leave me? I decided to enjoy the moment and see where it all led. One day at a time. But no more "comparison shopping" for the moment. I broached the subject of an exclusive relationship with Deborah and she agreed that we should give it a try.

One hundred eighty Minutes of Joy!!! Deborah surprised me with tickets to a Leonard Cohen concert and it was extraordinary. At the age of seventy-four, the "Bard of Montreal" still had a strong baritone voice and an incredible stage presence. He was backed by a talented eleven-piece band that played a variety of instruments.

My favourites were the riffs on the twelve string guitar, the mandolin, the stand-up bass, the saxophone and the harmonica. Because he is essentially a poet and his lyrics are so intense, his presentation of the hit songs that he has written was very much "poetry to music." Wonderful! It was best concert that I had ever attended.

As spring slowly emerged in Winnipeg, Deborah and I began to walk the linear park along the river in front of my house that extends for miles. It was great to get out and enjoy the weather, along with the dog walkers, cyclists and joggers.

I bought a bistro set and a new stainless steel barbeque for my sunroom, and Deborah and I enjoyed Sunday brunch *el fresco* before I left to visit Lynne and feed her lunch. Life, although complicated, was good.

I began to realize how happy I had become. I was seeing a lot of Deborah, and it was going well. As I got to know her better, I realized that although she and Lynne were quite different, they were similar in some important qualities.

Deborah could be very tough when she needed to (like Lynne), but she was very soft-hearted as well (again, like Lynne).

On one hand, Deborah was quite prepared to deal with staff that didn't measure up, and on the other, she went out and bought a new dress (out of her own pocket) for an elderly lady. She then persuaded a nurse's aide to do the woman's hair, so that she would feel pretty when she was discharged to a personal care home. The poor old girl had no family, but an abusive son to look after her.

Deborah's seven-year-old nephew, Devon, came over to visit and quite innocently put a lot of pressure on me. It was a rainy night, so Deborah brought sushi and we taught him how to eat with chopsticks. Then Devon and I played Battleship and checkers.

Devon had a great sense of humour and he took delight in referring to me as "Almost Uncle Tom"! He sat in my favourite leather chair, rocking back and forth and said man- to-man, "Almost Uncle Tom, when you and Aunt Deb get married, where are you going to live?" I said that I hadn't thought about it.

He then said, "No offence, Aunt Deb, but Tom's house is way cool! You should live here and give your house to David (my son)." We had a great time, and when we took him back to his grandma, he hugged me and said, "I love you, Tom." I hugged him back and told him that I loved him too! It just came out, as natural as can be. This was getting serious...

I visited with Lynne at noon on a Saturday, and then I drove up to Dauphin to meet Deborah and attend her family reunion dinner/reception. It worked out well, as I was able to go to the dinner and then a smaller breakfast (sixteen people) at Deborah's sister's farm the next morning. Then I went back to Winnipeg for dinner with Lynne.

I come from a small family, and boy—was that was an eye opener! Deborah's great grandpa emigrated from the Ukraine in 1898, and his brother came in 1914. There were over two hundred fifty people at the reunion, and only about half the family showed up.

I felt a little like a fish out of water, but everyone was very welcoming. Deborah had six siblings. Three brothers and three sisters. The oldest sibling (Lynda) had died of cancer. Running a farm and looking after a large family is a huge amount of work, so Deborah and her sister, Karen, who were close in age, were heavily involved in raising their younger siblings.

All of Deborah's brothers and sisters missed her greatly when she left home at eighteen. They adored her and she adored them. So I had to pass the sibling test. I think I received a strong recommendation from Devon (the nephew who I had entertained), who thought I was "way cool." It had been a while since I was subject to that type of scrutiny!

That fall, I asked Deborah to go on a couple of trips with me. I never went away for more than a week at a time because I worried a lot when I was away from Lynne. I had a very strong reason for making these trips as good as I possibly could for Deborah. Deborah was a cancer survivor. (That is my term. Deborah disagrees. She has told me in no uncertain terms that she *beat* cancer!)

Now, she informed me it was back. She was just diagnosed with breast cancer, again. Deborah's doctor detected it early, so the prognosis was good, but she was facing a mastectomy and possibly chemo.

Deborah asked me if I wanted to "check-out" of the relationship. I told her that I don't check-out" when the going gets tough, and that we could talk about our relationship after she was healthy again. She needed to have a positive outlook to beat this disease.

The first trip was to the east coast. I had always wanted to take a trip from Montreal to Halifax by train, to see the fall colours. And lo and behold, Via Rail had a sale! Just before we were to leave for Montreal, an early storm blew in, delaying our departure time from Winnipeg by three hours. This provided me an opportunity to visit Lynne and feed her lunch before we left. She was quiet and seemed tired. She still did well, but it seemed that her "off" days were a little worse than they used to be.

We flew to Montreal later in the day and spent the weekend downtown in old Montreal, at the Fairmont.

We then boarded the train in the Via station in Montreal, which happened to be under the Fairmont where we were staying. The train was called The Ocean, and the trip paralleled the St. Lawrence River from Montreal to Halifax. We left Montreal late on Monday and arrived in Halifax late on Tuesday.

We had a bedroom/shower on the train, with all meals included (the food is very good on Via), and guaranteed seating in the domed observation car to view the scenery and fall colours! They had docents in the car to explain the history and culture of the region as you rolled along.

We had champagne and wine tastings on the way in the dome car and then day trips along the east coast of Nova Scotia. We headed back to Winnipeg on Saturday.

The second trip I scheduled was to Florida in November, to just kick back, walk on the beach and enjoy fresh seafood. The Florida vacation was very laid back. We had a few nice dinners out, and I cooked up a few dinners of fresh fish in the condo.

The day usually involved a jog on the beach, followed by coffee/breakfast, overlooking the gulf. We had lunch in the same spot, another jog or we swam, and then a glass of wine while the sun was setting on the gulf. Then dinner. Hurricane Ida came through mid-week. It missed the gulf beaches, but we got some rain and high surf. We had lots of fun swimming in the waves.

I did get out to a large outlet mall south of Tampa and did some power shopping for Lynne at the Liz store with Deborah's help. Deborah was a saint. Great buys! Lynne was the consummate shopper and she would have been proud of us.

Deborah and I got back to Winnipeg in late November. The weather was incredible for that time of year! It was sunny and crisp—just above freezing with no snow, which is very unusual for November.

I went to visit Lynne as soon as we got back. She was quiet, but she gave me her little Mona Lisa smile and went, "Mmm!" when I hugged her. It made my day!

My doc had referred me to an urologist just before we left for Florida, because he suspected that I had prostate cancer, and I had a biopsy (a very unpleasant procedure!).

The urologist who performed my biopsy called me in late November on my return and told me that I had a small amount of cancer in one quadrant of my prostate. He told me that I would need a CT scan and a bone scan before meeting with him to discuss treatment options. In the interim, I would have a colonoscopy on December 14. Once all the tests were done, I would know what I was up against.

I gave Deborah the news that evening, and I told my son, Dave, on Sunday when he came over for Grey Cup. Everyone was very supportive. On a more positive note, Lynne was still making me smile. The high point for me was Lynne's Christmas party at Lion's on a Thursday, early in December.

I think that Lynne really enjoyed listening to the carols and nibbling on the treats that I fed her! I held her hands and moved them to the music while I sang along, and she seemed to like it. After all we've been through, she was still helping me through my day. Who would have thought... *Lord, I loved her!*

Deborah had a mastectomy and reconstructive surgery during the second week of December, 2009. I took Deborah in for surgery around five a.m. on a Friday. The operation lasted four hours, and she was out of intensive care and on the ward by about three p.m.

They told her that they would need to examine the tissue to determine what else needed to be done to treat the cancer. I asked Deborah to come and stay with me through the recovery period for the surgery (about a month) and she agreed.

I went out and bought a new bedroom suite and a flat screen TV for the master bedroom. I wanted Deborah to be as comfortable and happy as I could make her during her recovery period. I did have couple of worries about my ability to look after Deborah. One was my health. If I need surgery or treatment for cancer, I wouldn't be able to care for Deborah at the same time.

The other was Lynne. If Lynne were suddenly to take a turn for the worse, I wasn't certain that I could shoulder that burden and look after Deborah. Lynne was still my first priority. Deborah understood that she would need a "plan B" if either situation transpired.

None of this had been on my radar screen three months earlier, but I guess I had faced more difficult circumstances before, so I figured I'd get through this one. Lesson learned (or maybe re-learned)—live each day as though it may be your last. Enjoy life, give love and make a difference!

In the meantime I had a busy, stressful time preparing for the start-up of the $280 million Water Treatment Plant. Everything worked out, but I was exhausted.

I relaxed until Monday, when Deborah was discharged. Deborah's friends and co-workers began dropping off flowers, plants and food non-stop after she got out of the hospital. The house looked like a florist shop! Lots of *oohs* and *aahs* over the house, which was nice. It was just fine.

I just hid out in my office or went out to the garage to work on my Triumph. Deborah recovered well and had her drainage tubes removed later in the week. Her big watershed would be when she received the results of the tissue analysis and bone scan in early January. If the cancer had spread, things would be grim.

I had two doctor appointments and one procedure the week after Deborah was discharged, along with start-up and media relations for the largest project the city had ever built.

The procedure was a bone scan, which didn't hurt a bit. They gave me an injection of radio-active material (really, if you are travelling, they need to give you a letter, because you might set off radiation detectors) and I had to come back two hours later for the test. In between, I had to drink at least five glasses of water. The scan took about thirty minutes, while I was lying down. I fell asleep. Too much going on.

With that backdrop, I was on four different TV networks, as well as on a live radio interview and two newspaper interviews regarding the water treatment plant, going "live" the next day. *Man, did I look old on TV!* I just knew my son Dave would razz me!

On New Year's Eve, Deborah and I had a quiet night. I cooked us lobster and pasta in garlic and olive oil for dinner after I visited Lynne. Then I opened a bottle of champagne, and we watched the fireworks at the Forks from the front patio door. At midnight, I opened the front door to let the old year out and the New Year in, and we drank a toast to the future. And that year, I wasn't alone.

In early January of 2010, Lynne was still doing well, and as dear and lovable as ever. Deborah had healed well from her surgery and was soon scheduled to go back to work. So I thought, *What the heck?* and snagged us a sell-off for a five star all-inclusive in Mexico. Deborah had three doctors' appointments just before we left, and she would know the prognosis on her cancer fairly soon. It was something to keep our minds off an uncertain future.

We had a wonderful seven days in Mexico. We went to Los Cabos (we stayed at Riu Santé Fe) and had a great time. We took a day trip up about eighty miles north to a small town, where (apparently) the *Hotel California* in the Eagle's song was situated. Great shops and restaurants, and I ran into a guy (Gil Cloutier) whom I hadn't seen since grade six!

I had been in the paper a bit lately, and he recognized me. Good fun. We went whale watching and saw a thirty-five-foot, thirty-ton, grey whale, leaping out of the water like a pacific salmon. The best part about trip was swimming with the dolphins. What beautiful, intelligent creatures! It was wonderful.

When we returned from Mexico, Deborah received her oncology report from the surgery, and everything was good. The margins where clean and there was no evidence of cancer in the lymph nodes, so she didn't need chemotherapy. It was a great relief. She was happy, and so was I.

I met with another specialist (an oncologist) during the same week. We have the Prostate Cancer Center in Winnipeg, and he was one of the guys leading the charge there. He examined me and had blood taken for another PSA test. His strong recommendation was, "*Do Nothing.*"

He recommended blood tests every three months and biopsies every year, but in his view, the cancer was not likely to grow or spread quickly. Depending upon how things went and how old I was when the cancer became a risk, his recommendation was either nerve-sparing surgery or Brachytherapy.

The guy was an expert. I was very, very pleased and relieved. I would be around to keep my promise to Lynne. I would be there until the end.

Deborah was a very insightful woman. She knew immediately after we met that I wasn't ready to fully commit to a relationship, and she learned shortly thereafter that I didn't change very quickly.

But she was a patient woman and I guess she saw something in me that was worth waiting for. She once told me that I had walls around me and that she couldn't break them down. Only I could break down the walls and commit to loving her.

And so it was that the Universe, once again, helped me in an unexpected way. Deborah and I had been put through two terrible tests, our cancer diagnoses, and I finally had the strength to breach the walls. I finally let Deborah into my heart and the result was a feeling of pure joy. I told her that I loved her and I asked her to be my partner forever. She said, "Yes." And I love her dearly.

Parallel Lives

It has occurred to me that many of us live parallel lives, with not a lot of overlap between them. I have always maintained a degree of separation between my work and personal life. After Lynne got sick, work was something that I did to pay the bills. I worked to live rather than lived to work.

My true passion was caring for Lynne and doing my best to ensure her happiness. Things got a little muddled when I began to date, and even more so when I fell in love with Deborah. By then, I had three parallel lives!

Work remained my lowest priority. I had a fairly stressful job, with some significant responsibilities, but at the end of the day, it was just business. It wasn't that I didn't care about work. I just cared about Lynne and Deborah a whole lot more.

I loved Deborah and took delight in doing things that made her happy, but my commitment to Lynne was non-negotiable. I had promised Lynne that I would care for her to the end, and I intended to keep that promise. Fortunately for me, Deborah understood this completely. She was never jealous of the time that I spent visiting with Lynne, or of the restrictions that it placed on our schedule or how much I obviously loved Lynne.

I was fortunate to be able to come home from my visits with Lynne and discuss my experiences with Deborah. I could share the joy when things were good and share the pain and sorrow when they weren't. I was very fortunate to have this type of relationship with Deborah.

The next pages give you some snapshots of my parallel life with Lynne at Lion's. There were many ups and downs. Most of these snapshots are taken verbatim from emails to our friend Mary Sue. Mary Sue truly cared about Lynne and me and used to pray for us.

The early excerpts predate meeting Deborah. The fact that Deborah accepted Mary Sue and my friendship and accepted Mary Sue as her own friend speaks volumes about Deborah's character and her love for me. Many women would not have accepted Mary Sue's and my friendship. Deborah embraced it.

Jan 31, 2009

I usually visit Lynne at lunch time on weekends, instead of at dinner, and I just got home from our visit. She is having a great day. She overheard a couple of the little old ladies at the next table talking about, "what a nice young husband that poor girl has" (one of them is ninety-nine, and the other is one hundred and one!) and Lynne gave me a HUGE smile! I brought her a chocolate bar today, and told her she could only have it if she'd been a good girl. She giggled and said, "Well, I don't know!" We don't have many times like that anymore, and I've learned to treasure them.

Feb 1, 2009

I bought Lynne a box of Laura Secord creams (her favourite) today, and I'll pick up a card and flowers tomorrow, and take them to her at dinner time. It's our thirtieth wedding anniversary tomorrow! It seems like yesterday that she flashed that 1000 megawatt smile at me, and melted my heart! I KNOW she'll like the chocolates. She won't care about the card and flowers, but I will. Lord, I miss her! Tomorrow will be tough.

Feb 2, 2009

Lynne liked her chocolates, and she giggled when I read her card to her. I'm not certain whether she understood me, or whether it was just the inflection in my voice. I'd like to think that she understood, but that is likely just wishful thinking—and it doesn't matter. It's the smiles that matter.

They are tinkering with Lynne's medications right now. She has been crying out and shouting, and they wonder whether she might be in pain. She can't really communicate that sort of thing.

So they have stopped a medication designed to prevent osteoporosis (she is unlikely to survive long enough for that to be a problem) and have started a mild pain medication, to see whether that helps. She is always good with me. I think she somehow senses that I genuinely love her, and that comforts her. I wish that I could just hug her and draw all of the hurt out of her and into me!

Feb 8, 2009

Lynne is having ups and downs, but still has a lot of good days. I'm going to a "Sweetheart Luncheon" at Lion's with her this week. Lots of goodies. I'm sure Lynne will enjoy them!

Feb 10, 2009

Today was the "Sweetheart Luncheon!" Couples only! Of course, Lynne and I were the youngest in the room. Coincidentally, we were seated with a lady named Marylyn and her husband Bob. Marylyn and I attend the same Care Givers support group, so I know her well. She is well into her seventies, but very "spunky!" She lives in the Village, and wears red boots and has a colour coordinated red cane! Her husband is a delight, but very confused. But they were still able to have one dance together! Very heart warming.

They had live music (accordion; oldies like *Spanish Eyes!*), and served chicken Kiev and a very nice chocolate desert. Guess what Lynne liked! There were staff on hand to help feed Lynne, so I could actually eat, and spend time talking to her. I don't think that she understood what was going on, but she seemed to enjoy Bob's antics.

Feb 12, 2009

This will be a short email, as I'm on my way out the door, but I couldn't wait to tell you about this! I was very tired today, after two fairly adversarial meetings, and a conference call with our legal counsel all in one afternoon. So I almost skipped my visit with Lynne, so I could rest before another commitment this evening. At the last moment on my way home, I decided to stop and spend an hour with her.

Mary Sue, when I walked in, just for a moment, she knew me! She looked at me, said, "Oh!" and gave me the most beautiful smile! It was gone in an instant, but it lifted my spirits and brought tears to my eyes!

In your last email you said that you had prayed for Lynne and me. I think today, your prayers were answered. Thank you, Mary Sue.

Feb 16, 2009

Things I've learned; I have never said it out loud before, but for a while I was uncertain that I would be able to get through Lynne's tragedy in one piece (or maybe at all!). It has been very, very hard. But here I am. And I'm "sort of" whole.

I've learned that on some days, Lynne will be happy and smile, and on some days she won't. I've learned that it has nothing to do with me, and all I can do is my best. The days that she is good, I've learned to cherish. The days that she isn't, I've learned I can't change; all I can do is keep loving her, and wait for another good day. I also know that the time will come when there won't be any more good days. All the more reason to cherish them now.

Feb 19, 2009

Lynne is doing well. One of the nurses stopped by to chat while I was there tonight, and Lynne seemed to like seeing us talking together! She smiled and said, "Aw... that's nice!" and then chattered away in the cutest way! The nurse told me that Lynne seldom smiles for anyone but me! That made me smile, too!

Feb 20, 2009

When I went to visit Lynne on the way home today, she was a wee bit cranky! She doesn't talk any more in the conventional sense, but she was hollering at folks, and generally not a happy camper! I fed her dinner, and by then she was calm. I took her for a walk and talked to her, and by the time we were done, she was smiling!

We sat for a while in her room, and after a while I had her laughing and chattering away! Nothing that made any sense, but I haven't heard her laugh in a long time, and it was nice to hear it. I had planned to go out tonight, but decided to cancel. I wanted to sit and think about our life together, where we've been and where we are.

So I ate the last of the pasta from last Sunday (hopefully I'll survive that experiment!), drank a couple of glasses of red wine and some excellent single malt whiskey, listened to a favourite CD and reminisced. This one is for Lynne. It may seem sad, but it's not. It's full of good memories and hope.

30 Years

A beautiful smile
Flashing hazel eyes
Passion.
A lifetime begins
For two lovers.

Their destiny.

Happiness.
A child, now grown.
Ups and downs.
But love conquers
And love heals.
A good life, well lived.

Eyes that no longer flash,
But a smile that still moves me.
Love that no longer conquers
But still comforts
A good woman, well loved,
And heals her forever lover.

I realized today that I will always love Lynne, even after she is gone. But somehow she has given me permission to carry on. It's as though she has said, "It's OK; I want you to be happy! Just don't forget me!"

Feb 21, 2009

When I went to visit today, Lynne was sitting in her armchair, sound asleep. I sat on the arm of the chair and put my arm around her and kind of nuzzled up to her face, and she opened her eyes and said, "Yay!" very softly. It was wonderful. For some reason, cozy moments like that seem to trigger memories for her, especially if she is just waking up. Anyway, that's what made my day.

Feb 23, 2009

I found "Joy" in a surprising place, today. Lynne's table partner, Anne must be in her nineties, and lately she has stopped eating. I was afraid she had given up. She never seems to get any visitors, so I always make a point of saying hello, and giving her a smile when I sit down to feed Lynne. Today she had a sparkle in her eye when I said hello, and told me I looked very nice. She then looked at Lynne and said to her, "You must be his favourite girlfriend! Aren't you lucky?" Then she kind of chuckled. Very cute!

Author's Note: During the last bit of February and early March I was in Indian Wells at our time share; hence no emails about visits.

Mar 7, 2009

I went to see Lynne at lunch today, and I found myself eager to get there! For the first time since she became sick, I found myself missing her, just the way she is, and not way she used to be! On an emotional level, I've finally accepted her reality, and I missed not seeing her while I was away.

There is a huge difference between missing something and feeling guilty about it. When she first saw me, she got a little tear in her eye, and her lip trembled. I hugged her and kissed her forehead and patted her, and she smiled and was just fine. I had some tears of my own, but they were tears of joy!

Mar 24, 2009

Three Beautiful Words. Lynne was in fine form today! Lots of smiles and very vocal when I came to feed her dinner. Nothing that made any sense, but you could tell that she was happy. And afterwards, I had her laughing so hard that Maricel (one of the nurses) stopped by with a big smile to see what was up!

But here is what still has me a little teary. I put my arm around Lynne and said, "How did you get so cute!" and she giggled. Then I said, "Who's my girl?" and she grew very still. And then she said, very quietly, "I love you"! I never thought that I would hear her say those words again! If I die tomorrow, I will die a happy man.

Mar 29, 2009

Lynne is still doing well, and giving me sweet smiles when I visit. I had her hair done the other day, and the nurse on the floor made a point of telling me how hard it was for them to rinse the colour out of her hair. I guess it frightened her. It got me thinking.

Lynne always took great pride in her appearance, but I suppose that at this point, the colour only matters to me. So if it frightens her, no more colour! But it's going to be hard to watch my pretty girl go gray.

May 10, 2009

I went to visit with Lynne at noon, with bags full of gifts, cards, a birthday cake, ice cream, and plates and cutlery for her birthday party. After I fed her lunch, I spent a bit of time with her, reading her the cards from her brother Jack and I. I found the perfect card for Lynne! I couldn't have expressed my feelings any better if I have written it myself! The inscription read;

> "Happy Birthday
> To the Beauty of my days,
> The Joy of my world,
> The Love of my life."

When I read the card to her, Lynne took it from my hand, and looked at me and smiled! It was wonderful. David and Jackie arrived at 2:00 p.m. and we had a little birthday party for Lynne in the family room.

I bought Lynne a nice outfit (top, sweater and pants) from a European designer (Olsen) that Lynne used to be partial to, and some Purdy's chocolates that Deborah brought for me from Vancouver.

Lynne didn't seem to care much for the outfit (although it cost a fortune, I don't think she "understands" gifts much anymore), but she really liked the look of the chocolates! I sort of think of the outfit as being more for me than her, anyway. I know that she will look pretty in it, and that will make me happy.

She enjoyed the cake and candles, and our off-key rendition of *Happy Birthday!* When I left, Lynne was sitting in her chair in her room, quite content and dozing off.

Jun 6, 2009

When I visited Lynne today, I was late and missed her lunch (I broke a tooth at breakfast) and she was sound asleep. She looked like a little angel. I wished that I could put her in my pocket and take her home!

The swine flu is starting to be a bit of a worry here, and they are projecting that fifty percent of the population will be sick at some point. I worry about Lynne. She is doing well, and in good spirits, but is quite frail and I'm afraid that the flu might be too much for her.

I'm not ready to lose her. I love her far too much. I still visit her every day, and I miss her if I don't go. The other day, I patted the back of her neck while we watched TV, and she grew very still and had the nicest little smile on her face!

A Small Miracle: a couple of days ago after I fed Lynne and took her for a walk, we spent some time in her room watching TV, and as usual, I gave her hugs and told her I loved her, and that she was my girl! She understood me, and knew who I was, Mary Sue!

I looked down and she was sitting with her hands tightly clenched together, smiling, with trembling lips and tears running down her face. I knelt in front of her, and she looked at me lovingly and touched my face.

It only lasted a couple of minutes, but I will have it forever. God smiled on me. When I told Deborah about it, I couldn't keep the tears out of my eyes. She hugged me and told me that I was lucky to have two women that loved me! I guess I am.

Jul 21, 2009

I still see Lynne every day. She is still pleased to see me, and gives me a little smile when I come in, but she seems to be getting tired. She is very sleepy a lot of the time, and really has to work at walking, and I'm a little worried that she is beginning to decline. I know that this is inevitable, but I love her and I just hate to see it! She's still my girl, you know?

Jul 24, 2009

I had a nice visit with Lynne last night, with some laughs and cuddles, and we both left happy. She had seem tired a couple of days ago, and I was hopeful that with this improvement, things had turned around.

But I received a call from the nurse-practitioner early this morning, informing me that they had assessed Lynne recently, and that she was declining. Her brain can't properly command her legs to walk, and she likely will need to go into a wheelchair soon. The message (between the lines) is that she is comfortable, but things are going to get worse; a lot worse.

Lynne and I have been through this many, many times as she gets progressively worse, but it never seems to be any easier for me. Lord, how I hate that disease!

Lynne and my time together doesn't amount to a much anymore, but it is the best time we have left. It matters greatly, and I don't want to miss it. We need to live every day as though it is our last.

Aug 29, 2009

The other night at the end of our visit I said "Well, honey, I've got to go! It's almost seven p.m. and I haven't eaten dinner, and I'm hungry!" She looked at me, and made a funny face and said, "Aww," and then giggled. When I leaned over to give her a good-night kiss, she puckered up and then turned away and giggled some more. She was teasing me! Then I said, "I'll see you tomorrow night, and she smiled and said, "OK" and gave me a kiss.

Today, I went to visit her at lunch and she was laughing at the country music, and belting out notes! After lunch and a walk, I tried to leave a little early to get to another commitment, and she grew quite quiet and serious. I asked her if she would like it if I stayed a little longer, and she nodded. I stayed another 20 minutes (until my usual departure time) and then told her I'd see her tomorrow, and she smiled and gave me a good-bye kiss! It was well worth being late for an appointment!

It is impossible to know what is going on in her pretty head these days, but I need to believe that she still loves me and knows that I still love her! It's so important.

Aug 31, 2009

Lynne was in fine form today, although I'm going to have to buy her some chocolates! I brought a birthday card and some Laura Secord creams for Anne, her table partner. Anne turned 100 yesterday! Anyway, Lynne was looking longingly at the chocolates as we left the table, so I'll get her some in the next day or so. I think it's a gender thing. You women and chocolates! Anyway, Anne was delighted to get a little gift. She genuinely likes Lynne and me, and kind of watches out for Lynne. Isn't that ironic?

Sep 8, 2009

I've had three wonderful visits with Lynne in the last three days. I can't get much luckier than that! On Sunday, I visited Lynne at lunch time, and she dozed off with my arm around her while we watched TV. When she awoke, she opened her eyes and gave me the nicest smile, and nuzzled up against my chest!

It brought back some wonderful memories! Yesterday when I was feeding her dinner, she looked at me out of the blue, and said, "Well, Tom..." the way she used to when she would start to talk to me before she became ill. Of course, there was nothing else said, and it was a fleeting moment of lucidity, but that's OK. Today, she greeted me with a big smile and an "Oh!" uttered in a very pleased way. Very nice! I know that these are such small events, but they mean so much to me, and I treasure them.

Oct 3, 2009

One of the ladies (Julia) on Lynne's floor passed away last night. She was in her 90's, and always doted on Lynne when I walked Lynne by her table. Lynne seemed tired today, and looked at where Julia used to sit, as though she wondered where Julia had gone. I told her not to worry; Julia is happy in heaven. May God bless her! She was a kind old soul.

Oct 21, 2009

Lynne had a dental appointment and she always does better with me at her side, so I had to be at Lion's 1st thing. Lynne isn't used to seeing me in the morning, and she was quite happy and excited when she saw me! It was very sweet. More evidence that she knows me. And the dentist says "No cavities!" A good outcome.

Dec 5, 2009

Lynne is almost like having a grandchild now. I sit with her and tell her she's a good girl, give her hugs and stroke her hair. She laps it up. She has this little smile I call her "Mona Lisa" smile while this is going on. It reminds me of when I used to hold Dave when he was a baby. It is very special.

Dec 30, 2009

Lynne is doing well, but I think that she is starting to slow down, Mary Sue. I doubt that she will be walking by the end of next year, and after that, complications are likely to set in. But I still go every day, and she still walks for me and seems to like it when I stroke her ear or her cheek. When I give her a kiss and say, "Mmm," while I hug her, she often says, "Mmm," back!

Feb 2, 2010

Today is Lynne and my thirty-first wedding anniversary. It's strange how you think that something like that won't affect you, and then it wallops you like a rogue wave at the beach. I found myself lying awake last night, thinking about times gone by and maybe weeping a bit. It's a good thing that Deborah sleeps soundly.

Today I'll take Lynne a card and some Laura Secord truffles, and a red rose. She won't understand the card or the rose, but it won't matter. They are in a way, for me. She will enjoy the chocolates. I'll feed her a chocolate or two, show her the flower and read the card to her. Then I'll give her some hugs, and make sure she doesn't see me cry.

This is her poem:

Lynne

She no longer speaks.
She can barely walk.
But she still smiles
Now and then.
And it lights up the room.
Time has pared her
Down to the barest essence
Of who she was...
She is gentle.
She is kind.
She has more courage
Than anyone should ever need.
And she needs love to live.
So I give it to her.
A gentle touch
A soothing voice
Caring arms.
For my beautiful wife.

31 years

Mar 7, 2010

Well, our week in Palm Springs was over in a blink! When I went to visit Lynne at lunch on Saturday, she was waiting quietly for the food to arrive in her chair in the cafeteria. When I sat next to her she looked a little vacant to me. Then I said, "Hi Sweetie!" and she looked at me and teared up and gave a little sob!

I said, "Did you miss me Hon?" and she said, "Yaa!" I gave her hugs and patted her hands and back and all was well. Today, everything was back to normal when I went to visit.

Mary Sue, she must have loved me more than I can imagine, for her to still remember after all this time. I suppose that most people would not consider me particularly fortunate, given Lynne's trials and my own health issues, but I am a very lucky man.

Apr 3, 2010

Today when I arrive to feed Lynne lunch, she was still lying on bed after her morning nap. I went over and said, "Hello" and she said, "Oh!!!" and got all excited! I put her shoes on, and brushed her hair and put her glasses on and asked if I could take her to lunch. She began to laugh and chatter and broke out into a huge smile! God's Easter gift to me. It was truly wonderful.

Apr 24, 2010

After I feed Lynne her meal, I take her for a little walk to the end of the hall. There is a small sun room there, and we stand together and I tell her what it's like outside, and point out the people and traffic on the street.

We were standing there in the afternoon sun yesterday, and she looked at me and said, "Mine!!!" I looked at her and said, "Yes Honey, I'm yours and your mine. I love you very much." She gave me her little "Mona Lisa" smile, and we went to finish her walk, before she got too tired from standing. It was a beautiful moment.

May 10, 2010

My son Dave and his wife Jackie met me at Lion's today, to celebrate Lynne's sixty-second birthday. She was napping when I arrived, and when I woke her she was so excited to see me! She was smiling and laughing and chattering away! All the healthcare folks had to smile when they saw her like that! I brought a Jeanie's Bakery cake (a family tradition) and ice cream, and her gifts, and we had a little party in the family room. It was great!

I still love her, Mary Sue. And I think she still loves me!

May 11, 2010

I forgot to tell you a little story about birthday cards. Sort of funny, but pretty embarrassing at the time! When I went to buy Lynne's card, I realized that Deborah's birthday was also coming up in May, so I bought her a card as well… When I went up to the cashier at Safeway to pay, the lady looked over the two cards. One read "Happy Birthday to my Lovely Wife" and the other read "Happy Birthday to my Sweetheart."

Mary Sue, she gave me a withering look that placed me firmly in the same category as pond scum! She thought that I was cheating on my wife. I just looked at her and said, "It's complicated!" and walked out! I'm certain that she went home and told her friends and family about the low life she encountered at work! Walk a mile in my shoes—my buddies thought it was pretty funny—I suppose it is. Sort of.

Lynne was tired tonight, but wanted to cuddle up while she snoozed. In a way, she is like the granddaughter I wish I had. So sweet. It was pretty neat.

May 30, 2010

I got Lynne some new clothes at the Liz outlet store when we were in Minneapolis. She always liked to look for bargains on designer stuff, so I thought I'd continue the tradition! Anyway, the staff at Lion's has been dressing her up like a little doll! Black track suit with a red top and red Sketchers! Or blue with blue Sketchers, etc. It's nice to see her looking the way she would have liked to, if she were able.

When I went to see her the other day, she was sitting in her room. When I arrived, she was very pleased to see me. She chattered and laughed, and when we went out for lunch, she had a great big smile on her face, which made the staff smile as well.

That's the good part of a day when she has improved cognitive ability—the bad part is when I sat her down for lunch, and she surveyed her surroundings. Then she became upset and agitated. You could see it in her eyes. If she could speak, she would have said, "What am I doing here with all these old people?"

It's strange how you can have a magic moment and one that is intensely sad within a period of five minutes. But you just need to count the magic moments as a blessing, and live with the sadness. The sadness never really goes away. But neither does the love! That's what keeps me going, Mary Sue. The love. It really does conquer all.

Jun 5, 2010

When I went to visit Lynne at lunch today, she was as perky as can be! All smiles and chattering away when I entered her room. When I took her for lunch, she became a little quiet and held my hand tightly while I fed her. Bon Jovi came on the radio with, *Do You Want to Make a Memory*, and Lynne seemed to be listening to it. I said, "We have a lot of memories, don't we Sweetie?" and she said, very seriously, "Uh huh!" and nodded. Mary Sue, it was all I could do to hold back the tears.

Jul 4, 2010

Lynne has had ups and downs the last week or so. One day she was puffing and could hardly walk, and the next she seemed OK. She was very quiet and didn't seem to know me early in the week, which always makes me feel very sad.

Then today, she was perky as can be and greeted me with a big smile and chattered away to me!

She did one thing that really tugged at me heart strings! While I was feeding her, she said, "Like you!" I said, "I love you too, Honey!" Then she said, "Always?" And I said, "Yes Honey, I will love you forever!" Mary Sue, I don't know whether she really says what I think she is saying, or understands me, but I need to believe that she does. It's a little like faith.

Jul 12, 2010

I had a wonderful moment with Lynne on Saturday. She was very happy to see me and laughed and chattered when I came to get her for lunch. But the best part came after I fed her and was taking her for a walk. I always walk backwards ahead of her so that I can hold her hands and lead her forward. She never looks at me while I am doing this; she just kind of gazes off into space. Mary Sue, this time she looked me in the eye and gave me the nicest little smile! It was the smile she used to give me that said "I love you!" I am certain that at that instant, she knew me. A magic moment. And truly one to remember.

Aug 1, 2010

I've been battling a cold all week. Every day I would go to work, come home for a nap at noon, and still have no energy at all left by the end of the day. I was far too tired to visit Lynne, and didn't want her to catch what I had anyway!! So I missed seeing her for the whole week, until Saturday, when I started to feel a bit better...

When I arrived on Saturday she was sitting in the dining room waiting for lunch. I sat with her and talked and held her hands, and she grew very excited and began to laugh and smile! It made my week, because I had been missing her so much! Mary Sue, I think that the most precious gift God has bestowed on me is the ability to make my girl smile! I truly treasure it!

Aug 8, 2010

Ann (Lynne's table partner at meals) passed away on Saturday. Ann was a dear old girl who just turned 100 this year. She always had a smile and a wave for me, and believe it or not, she kind of watched out for Lynne. I asked God to welcome her in heaven, and I asked Ann to "learn the ropes" so she could help Lynne when her time comes.

Aug 10, 2010

Today was the best visit that I can recall having with Lynne since she went into care almost two years ago. She was very alert; smiling and laughing a lot, and looking at what was going on around her with great curiosity!

After I fed her dinner, we had our usual walk and then sat in her room and watched TV. That's the normal routine. But she started chirping away at me in a very animated way, so I laughed and said, "What?" to her. She laughed back and said, as clear as can be, "I don't know!"

Mary Sue, Lynne hasn't uttered an entire sentence in a long, long time! She seemed to understand everything that I was telling her. I took her hands and sang to her while moving her hands to the music of a song on TV, and she laughed and laughed! Then she clapped her hands as though applauding!

Even though I was dead tired (I had meetings all day and missed lunch) I stayed a little longer than usual because I didn't want to miss the magic! When I did tell Lynne I needed to go she grew quiet and solemn. I asked her if she would like me to stay a while longer and she said, "YES!" and nodded her head.

When I did finally go, I told her I would be back tomorrow, "same time and same place". She said, "OK!" and I gave her a hug and a kiss and left her smiling quietly. It was all very wonderful. She was such a dear!

Mary Sue, I know that I can't hope for many more days like this one, but I felt blessed today. Today, life was truly amazing! I smiled all the way home.

I plan to talk to the nurse and find out whether there have been any changes to Lynne's meds. She stopped getting the usual drugs for Alzheimer's about four years ago. They were no longer helping and they had some adverse side-effects. Could she be getting better? That would be a miracle, and I can't allow myself to hope for a miracle. Been there, done that... It is just too painful.

Aug 19, 2010

Pure Happiness! On Saturday when I went to visit Lynne, she was still in bed having a morning nap. The health care aid said that she would look after getting her up, but I told her I didn't mind doing it. When I leaned over to give Lynne a hug and a smooch, she beamed and said, "Aww, I like him! " Needless to say, those words made my day! She was all smiles, until I put her shoes on her feet.

When I put her shoes on, Lynne became a little cranky and said, "SHIT!" I couldn't see anything wrong, so I got her up and took her for a little walk, after which she seemed a little happier. Then I looked down and realized that I had placed her shoes on the wrong feet! I switched them around and Lynne was much happier! But she did give me the "You dumb *shmuck*" look! Oops!

Sep 12, 2010

The beginning of the week was pretty grim for me, Mary Sue. Lynne was having terrible difficulty walking, and didn't seem to know me at all. It broke my heart to see her trying so hard to will her legs to take each step. And when she looked at me there was no glimmer of recognition—no light in her eyes—so I had a little talk with myself and decided that it didn't matter whether she knew me or not; what mattered was that I knew who she was.

When you remember how much love someone has brought into your life, it is easy to be there for them and to give them love back, whether they know it or not. One of the health care aids came up to me while I was feeding Lynne and said, "You know, she can feel the love when you hold her hands." I hope that is true. It's very important to me.

Later in the week, Lynne improved and now she seems to be her old self, at least for a while! She is walking better and chattered at me today when I went to see her. She was so cute! One of the staff was giving another resident what-for for something she shouldn't have done, and Lynne smiled and said, "Uh oh!" So I have my girl back for a while.

Deborah is working much too hard right now. She can't say no to people that need her, and I worry about how tired she is sometimes. So I give her "the talk" and take her out for dinner and that seems to help.

September 23, 2010

Deborah and I celebrated my fifty-ninth yesterday, and it was a great day. Deborah bought me a case of wine and PJs, and took me to Amici's for dinner. Very nice!

Lynne, in her own way also gave me a wonderful gift— she was very vocal and chattered away to me! I didn't know what she was saying, and I'm pretty sure she didn't understand me, but she did understand the hugs and kisses, and we both understood the smiles and laughter. It was a day to treasure and remember.

My gift to myself was a train ride through the Rockies. We fly to Edmonton today and catch the train early tomorrow a.m. We're travelling deluxe in a bedroom car, meals and access to the Park Car (dome car) included. It should be fun. Then we'll spend a few days in Vancouver visiting with friends and family, and come back on Tuesday.

Oct 12, 2010

We got back to Winnipeg on Tuesday and when I visited Lynne on Tuesday evening, her face lit up and she began to laugh and chatter at me! What a wonderful homecoming! I honestly believe that there are times when she still knows me and remembers that she loves me.

Those moments are very precious to me. I am a very lucky man. She has been very happy for the last 10 days or so, and gives me a big smile and an "Aww" when I give her a hug and a kiss. I bought her some souvenir T-shirts and some Purdy's chocolates in Vancouver, and she has been gobbling up the chocolates.

Oct 30, 2010

Deborah works very long hours sometimes, and the nature of the work (helping people who are under duress due to health or emotional problems) can be stressful. So I worry about the impact on her health. Every now and then I have to remind her that there are more important things than work! And that she can't help everyone! (This coming from a reformed workaholic!)

Nov 1, 2010

I'm waiting for my hero to come home from work. There was a serious car accident last night, involving three young girls. They were broadsided by another young girl who was under the influence and ran a red light at sixty mph. One of the girls died on the way to the hospital. The second died this afternoon in emergency.

The third, who was driving, is critical, but stable. Deborah had to tell her that her two close friends didn't make it, so now the poor girl, in addition to dealing with her own injuries must cope with the grief of losing her friends.

The only luck this young girl has had in the last day is Deborah. Deborah is very good at what she does, and I know she will help her through. For my part, I'll make Deborah a nice dinner and pour her some wine, and listen to her talk...

Yes, I'm proud of her!

Dec 5, 2010

Sorry I haven't been keeping up with news, but my back has been against the wall a little at work, keeping up with the lawyers on the Veolia contract. I've been working every night, as well as attending Lynne's year end care conference and molly-codling Deborah.

Deborah just had surgery on December 2. Part two of the reconstructive procedure that began with her mastectomy last year. She is doing well, and I'm taking her to Florida on Tuesday to recover for a week or so at the beach.

The Lion's staff at the care conference told me that they were amazed how well Lynne is doing. That doesn't mean she is getting better, Mary Sue. She is still slowly getting worse. But she is doing much better than expected, and they think that it is partly because of me.

Supporting Lynne is the most important thing I do. The other day when I arrived Lynne was still having a nap, and I gently woke her up for lunch. She was so excited and happy! I said, "Are you happy to see me?" and she said, "Really, really!"

A wonderful moment. I took her to the Lion's Christmas concert on Dec 2. She was a little apprehensive at first (lots of people and noise), but I held her hands and sang along to the Christmas carols to her, and she liked it.

That was a long day! I drove Deborah for her surgery at seven-fifteen a.m., worked till noon, brought Deborah home and made her lunch, worked in my home office while keeping an eye on Deborah until five p.m., went and fed Lynne and took her to the concert, arrived home at eight-thirty p.m., cooked dinner and collapsed! Yikes!

I filed my retirement paperwork this Friday! My last day on the payroll will be January 14, 2011. But I've agreed to work on contract until the end of June, four days a week. After that I'm going to take the summer off, and I'm not sure whether I'll go back.

I kind of think that June will be the end. Mary Sue, you have no idea how free I felt when I dropped off those papers! Next summer I'll be cycling, kayaking and driving my old car instead of going to the office! *Yahoo!*

Dec 24, 2010

I've been quite ill with the flu, almost from the time the plane touched down from Florida—high fever (101 or 102) coupled with a screaming headache, cough and "achy" all over, and wake up soaked in sweat every morning! The worst part of it is that it has put me off my two favourite beverages on the planet—coffee and red wine!

I had a wonderful visit with Lynne on our return (all smiles, chattered away at me and actually planted a kiss on my cheek when I hugged her!), but haven't gone since because I didn't have the energy, and I was afraid she might catch it!

For some reason, Deborah didn't get it from me (thank goodness!). Deborah has been taking good care of me. It feels a little strange (but really nice) to me to be on the receiving end, after being a caregiver for so long...

I started on an anti-viral medication two days ago, and I'm finally starting to feel better, so I'm on my way to see

Lynne right after I finish writing to you. I haven't been able to rest as much as I would have liked to due to work demands, but am now looking forward to a four and a half day stretch to rest up, as much as I can with six dinner guests tomorrow and fourteen on Boxing Day (yikes!).

Christmas is always a little bittersweet for me. I have all these memories of our family with Lynne, and I tend to miss her terribly. It's nice to have a new family to entertain at Christmas, made up of Deborah's and mine. I have one tradition that I plan to keep up for Lynne, for as long as I am on this earth.

Lynne used to nag me unmercifully until I made two donations at Christmas, one to the Christmas Cheer Board, for toys and hampers to needy families, and one to Winnipeg Harvest, to provide food to families in need.

In Lynne's mind, the first was for the children's souls, and the second was for their tummies. So every year I drive to the Free Press building (the local paper coordinates the drive) and drop off two cheques for $250 each with a note explaining the history of the donation, and that when they recognize donors on the newspaper, this one should just say "for Lynne."

This year the reporter who looks after the fund raising drive must have opened the letter just I was walking out the door. He ran out into the parking lot to tell me my story was very moving and to thank me for the donation. I told him that he should thank my lovely wife, who can no longer speak on her own behalf. This is her legacy.

Jan 1, 2011

Lynne remains happy and gives me a smile when I visit, but she is refusing to eat. She hasn't had any solid food for about 10 days, and I'm worried, Mary Sue. When I visited her yesterday, it took me an hour to feed her an energy shake and a bowl of soup.

She has lost some weight and is have difficulty standing and walking because she is getting weak. After our walk, she just plops down in her chair and dozes off, with my arm around her and her head on my shoulder. That's when the tears come—I hope that it is just a bug, and she'll pull out of it. I'm not ready to let her go.

During our last care conference, the social worker at Lion's reminded me that I had not made funeral arrangements for Lynne (they asked me to do it 2 years ago), and said it would be a lot easier now than when Lynne passes.

Deborah, who has had to look after arrangements for both her father and her sister is also telling me "get it done!" so I guess I will, in January. I don't want to, though. Say a prayer for Lynne, Mary Sue. I already have, but I think that you are a lot closer to God than I.

I am retiring on January 14, and will start work on contract on Jan 17, four days a week until July 1. Then who knows? I'm going to use that extra day to work on my cars, visit Lynne and work out.

Jan 19, 2011

I'm sitting in my red leather rocker with the ottoman, drinking coffee and looking out at the trees and the river. Winter here is quite beautiful, if you know where to look. It is supposed to be a little warmer here today, so I'll clear the walk after visiting Lynne.

I had a short snooze yesterday afternoon, and I dreamt that Lynne had passed on and I was telling Dave what a wonderful mother she had been for him. I woke up with tears running down my face, to hugs from Deborah. Life is full of ironies. Thank God I have people close to me to see me through this next trial, and give me courage so that I can see Lynne through it as well.

Jan 20, 2011

Lynne hasn't eaten any solid food since mid-December. She can still walk, but not as far as she used to. She seems to be in some pain. She is so brave, Mary Sue! She sits and moans a bit because she is hurting, but she still has a smile and a little coo for me when I give her a hug! But seeing her like that makes me very, very sad.

With Deborah's help, I've worked out the details of her funeral, although I have not yet finalized the arrangements. It was hard to do. It seemed like I was giving up on Lynne, in a way. I'm not, though. I'll be there for my girl for as long as we are both on this earth.

February 2 will be Lynne and my thirty-second wedding anniversary. And her twelfth year with Alzheimer's. Lynne looked after me for 21 years, and I've looked after her for 12. My privilege and duty. I took those vows very seriously.

Jan 30, 2011

As you know, Lynne hasn't been doing very well. Mary Sue, on Thursday and Friday she chattered away at me, all smiles and laughter! On Friday I tickled her tummy and she giggled and said, "No, no, no!" and laughed! On Saturday she was tired.

Now and then she lies awake all night. No one knows why. Today she was in fine form and actually said my name! She seems happy. I know that it won't last forever, but I will gladly take whatever joy Lynne can provide!

One of the staff at Lion's told me that I was a very devoted husband and that she believed that Lynne still knew the sound of my voice and my touch. She said that Lynne lived for me. I was moved by those kind words.

Feb 2, 2011

Well, Lynne gave me my anniversary gift a day early.
Last night, she was just a sweetheart! She smiled and
laughed and talked up a storm! She would chatter away and
then pause and I'd say, "OK!" Then she'd say, "Well, OK!"
and chatter some more. Very dear. I usually give Lynne a
little hug after our walk, before I sit her down. Last night
she hugged me back and gave me a pat on the back and a
little peck on the cheek! A wonderful visit.

Tonight, Lynne was a little tired. I usually buy her
chocolates, but I didn't this year (she won't eat them
anymore). It seemed like a loss of sorts to me. Lynne loved
chocolates as much as you do! I bought her a nice card and
some red roses. She used to love red roses. But now she
doesn't understand what the roses are, or what I was saying
when I read the card to her. I suppose the whole thing is
more for me than for Lynne.

But you know something, Mary Sue? I think in her way
Lynne still loves me, and I know that I still love her. And
that's worth celebrating. Right?

Feb 6, 2011

Yesterday when I went to see Lynne, she was laying in
her bed crying. I asked her what was wrong, and of course
she couldn't tell me. When I tried to hug her, she shrank
away as if she was afraid! Of course, this brought tears to
my eyes, but I kept trying to reassure her, and eventually
she was OK.

I think maybe she'd had a bad dream. I put her shoes
on her feet, and sat her up and brushed her hair. And
hugged her some more. By the time I walked her out for
lunch she was calm. By the end of lunch she was smiling
quietly.

When I got home, Deborah asked me how Lynne had
been. I said, "OK." Deborah told me to sit down and tell her

the real story, which I did. This resulted in more hugs, this time from Deborah.

Today, when I visited Lynne, she was quite perky and verbal. She chattered away at me and I talked to her. And now and then we would share a laugh! And I thought, *Lynne can't understand much of what I say, and I don't know what she is trying to tell me, but I still know what she is feeling!*

And then it occurred to me. Lynne, Deborah and I all share the same language: *it is the language of love.*

Feb 10, 2011

Today I slipped away from the meetings for a very important luncheon engagement. It was the Valentine's Day lunch at Lion's. When I arrived, Lynne was already down in the common room. And she was in tears. The noise and different surroundings were too much for her. When I snuggled her, she would stop sobbing, but as soon as I stopped, the tears started again.

So I took her back up to her floor. The staff (very graciously) followed with both our meals, and seated us in one of the private family rooms, with roses and romantic music!

Mary Sue, it was so cute! Lynne stopped crying and sort of looked around and got this great big smile on her face! It was as though she thought *This looks pretty good!* She laughed and chattered to me, and when I asked her if she was my Valentine, she giggled and said, "OK!" It truly made my day!

Feb 12, 2011
Deals you make with God

Thanks for the email yesterday. What I do for Lynne is as much for me as for her. It's all about love. And promises to keep. I'm going to tell you about some folks I saw yesterday, and then write about what was going through my mind just before my by-pass surgery, and I think that you will understand.

Yesterday, Deborah and I went to cancer-care for my three month check-up. My PSA was up a bit from last time, but not enough to cause any real worries. The Doc is going to schedule me for another biopsy in April, and then we'll see.

It is always a bit of a worry, and sometimes I fret about it. That was all put into perspective with what Deborah and I saw as we got onto the elevator to leave the building. It is an image that has been haunting me ever since.

When we got on the elevator there was a young couple holding their 18 month old daughter. Emily. She had cancer. She was bald, lethargic and had a port attached to her arm for her medications, which she had just received. She wasn't crying. She was smiling and trying to be brave for her parents' sake.

And her parents were smiling and trying to comfort her, but the hurt in their eyes was palpable. I thought to myself *So many tears. There must be so many tears in that home.* And so many "Deals you make with God." Any parent would offer up the prayer, "Take me and spare my child!" I know, given the choice, that I would. Deborah and I left with tears in our eyes, counting our blessings.

But it reminded me of a deal that I had proposed, just before my by-pass surgery. My prayer went, "Please Lord, let me live so that I can care for Lynne for as long as she may live." I wasn't afraid of death, I was afraid of leaving Lynne when she needed me.

Lynne once asked me, early on in her illness, "What will happen to me?" And I told her that I would be there to love her and care for her forever. She said, "To the end? Promise?" and I said, "Yes, dear, I promise." That was an important moment for Lynne, because while we had our disagreements (every couple does) I had never broken a promise to Lynne. After that, Lynne didn't dwell on being sick because she knew I would care for her.

So looking after Lynne is about love, and keeping a promise. And maybe a deal I struck just before my surgery.

Author's Note: Some readers may wonder why there is such a large gap (about a month) between the above email and the next one. The simple explanation is that Deborah and I were in Indian Wells for ten days in late February arranging renovations to our condo, and we updated Mary Sue concerning Lynne while we were there.

Mar 14, 2011

I went to visit Lynne yesterday and she was alternately weeping uncontrollably and angry the whole time, with two small periods where she seemed to know me and smiled and laughed. I spoke to the nursing staff and they told me that Lynne wasn't sleeping at all and that they have prescribed *triazadone* (a mild antidepressant) to help her sleep and hopefully cheer her up.

They aren't sure what has caused the change in behaviour. Apparently it has been going on for about a week. Of course, I worry that I was away too long, and Lynne might be doing better if I had been here.

It broke my heart to see Lynne that way, Mary Sue. I stayed with her for two hours, and she cried most of the time. I tried hugging her and talking to her and kissing her, but nothing helped! When I left, I broke down and cried in the car. I was exhausted.

Deborah has tried to reassure me that it wasn't my being away that caused this; just the progression of the disease. But I'm not certain of that. It doesn't really matter anyway. This isn't about me. It's about my Lynne. I'll suck it up and do all that I can to make her feel better. Say a prayer for her, Mary Sue! She may need more help than I can provide. I can't bear to see her so unhappy.

Mar 15, 2011

Lynne knew me when I went yesterday! She is very tired from not sleeping; with dark rings under her eyes and quite thin. But there was no crying! Oni (one of the rec coordinators) likes Lynne a lot and was feeding her when I arrived.

Lynne looked right at me in an inquiring way, laughed, and began chattering! After I walked her back to the room, I sat her in her chair and gave her hugs and talked to her. I need to kneel on the floor in front of her now to make eye contact, because her head droops forward. Another "benefit" of Alzheimer's.

She was able to form some words, and said, "Don't go wa(y?)" and then proceeded to chatter at me angrily, as though she was giving me what-for for being away too long! I think my prayers have been answered! We'll see how she is today.

I spoke with the nurse practitioner (Preta) after our visit, to discuss Lynne's condition and the drug dose. She said that now that I am back, Lynne may do better, in which case they can reduce the *triazadone* dose. But for now, the priority is for Lynne to get more sleep.

I told Preta that I had never left Lynne for more than a week, and I felt guilty because my absence likely hurt Lynne. Preta said, "Some people don't believe in this, but I think that people with serious dementia still remember the people that they love. It's deep inside of them. Lynne must have loved you very much. Your daily visits make a great difference in her, but you must look after yourself, so that you can continue to care for Lynne."

So that is what I will do. Balance, right Mary Sue?

My other girl now has us on a healthy meal regimen and is working out every day at the Refit gym. I told her that if she didn't stop working so hard and begin to look after herself, I might end up looking after her too! Once Deborah puts her mind to something, it happens!

Deborah is counselling a young woman who experienced a tragic loss right now. She loves helping young people, and seems to make a real difference to them. I've seen a young woman come up to Deborah in a shop and thank her for turning her life around. Powerful stuff! I told Deborah that once she retires, she should keep up her private practise if she finds it rewarding. She said, "Looking after you is a full time job!" We'll see.

From Mary Sue:

Please don't feel guilty. You count too. God knows you have and are doing a superior job with Lynne—you were the best husband for all those years—and continue to be. Do not feel guilty about Deborah—did you read that???? Do not feel guilty about Deborah...I believe she was sent to you and you deserve her. Please get rest yourself, OK—and give my best to Deborah and hugs to Lynne.

Mar 16, 2011

Yesterday, Lynne had some good moments while I fed her dinner, and walked her, and then about thirty minutes of non-stop sobbing with a few moments of laughter while I sat with her in her room. I am convinced now that the erratic behaviour is due to the progression of the disease.

It breaks my heart to see her this way. When I hold her she hugs me very tightly, like a small child, but she won't stop sobbing. They plan to increase her meds today, and maybe that will make a difference.

After visiting her, I had a dynamite tension headache, but I didn't cry this time! And a couple of glasses of wine and a nap helped the headache. All I can do is be there to comfort her as best I can, and advocate on her behalf to ensure that she is getting the right meds.

If things don't improve soon, I'll get in touch with her old specialist, Dr. Campbell, and ask him for some advice on treatment.

And yes, Mary Sue, she still knows me. I can see it in her eyes when she looks at me, and feel it when we hug. And I think that she knows that I love her. When she was crying and difficult, I told her that it didn't matter what she did, I would never stop loving her and being there for her. She could always count on her Tommy. She just pressed her face more tightly against mine, and kept on sobbing. But she understood.

Mar 18, 2011

Lynne isn't doing well, Mary Sue. She no longer cries, but I think that she is over-medicated. She is very passive, tired and is having trouble swallowing. She isn't distressed, but she doesn't experience any joy.

I am afraid that she will aspirate some of her food while eating and get a lung infection. In her weakened state I doubt that she would survive that type of infection. I'll give it a couple of days and then speak to the health care professionals. At least she isn't distressed. But I miss the spark between us.

Mar 22, 2011

Lynne is having ups and downs. She had a couple of days where she almost seemed to be in a trance. Very calm, but very little emotion. I spoke to the charge nurse over the weekend, and she said that Lynne still wasn't sleeping through the night. The nurse (Sharon) said that perhaps Lynne's sleep patterns were messed up.

Sharon said that when she was on nights Lynne was calling out. Sharon went to see whether she could calm her down. Sharon asked Lynne if she wanted to go for a walk and Lynne said, eagerly, "OK!" So they walked until Lynne was tired. It doesn't take very long to tire her out, these days.

Sharon put her back to bed with the teddy bear that my son Dave got her, and she started to drift back to sleep. But when Sharon tried to leave, Lynne's hand shot out and clutched Sharon's arm. She held her there until she went to sleep. Like a little girl.

It helps a great deal that the staff at Lion's express genuine affection for Lynne and provide (I believe) the best care possible. Mary Sue, you have no idea how many places I visited before I chose Lion's for Lynne. Thank goodness I did my homework. It is, after all, her final home.

The next day, while I was feeding Lynne her lunch one of the nurses came by to give Lynne her meds, and Lynne wouldn't take them. The nurse asked me to try, and Lynne took them immediately. Of course, this caused the nurse and Paula, the health care aide who was feeding Ruth across the table from us to tease Lynne. "Oh, you won't do it for us, but you will for Tom!"

This caused me to tell them a story that I've likely told you as well. It's one of those wonderful memories that I carry in my heart. When Lynne and I lived in our big house in the burbs, I always helped Lynne down the stairs from her bedroom, while Wendy or Janet from Home Care waited in the breakfast nook.

The stair from the second story came down into the living room, to a landing about six feet above the floor and then made a right angle turn towards the rear of the house. Lynne would always stop dead in her tracks at the landing, and she wouldn't move until I gave her a kiss on the cheek! This would always bring a smile from the ladies that were looking after Lynne while I went to work.

Lynne sat quietly in her little trance while I told the story, and I didn't think that she understood what I was saying. Then Paula said, "Look at Lynne!" Mary Sue, she was sitting there with the nicest smile on her face! I guess Lynne and I both share that memory, or perhaps Lynne was reacting to the love she hears in my voice when I tell the story.

The day after, the charge nurse informed me that pharmacist and nurse practitioner had consulted and they adjusted Lynne's meds yet again. They left the evening dose of *triazadone* in place to help Lynne sleep, eliminated the morning dose of *triazadone* to keep her alert during the day, and increased her daily pain meds.

They believe that she may be calling out because she is pain, but they've checked her out and can't find any obvious causes. I think that they may be on the right track. When I visited Lynne at noon yesterday, Lynne was calling out and distressed. After her pain med, she was quite calm. It is so hard to know what might be the right thing to do, because Lynne cannot speak.

Lynne had a health care directive drafted by our family lawyer after she was diagnosed with Alzheimer's, while she was still competent. She did not want me burdened with treatment decisions as the disease progressed. She was adamant that the only treatment she wanted was whatever was needed to keep her comfortable until she passed on. So that is what we will do.

Mary Sue, when I see Lynne in pain or distressed, it breaks my heart! Deborah listens patiently, asks all the right questions and then helps me to resolve my emotions. She must get tired of hearing about it, but it never shows.

And when the time is right, she will arrange for dinner with friends or a concert so we have some good times to offset the painful ones that I've been facing. It's as though I have my own live-in therapist/entertainment director (who loves me a great deal) to help me through my days!

Our relationship is one of mutual love, respect and support. Although these days, I feel as though I've been taking more than giving. And then you put up with these long, meandering emails. I am truly a lucky man!

Mar 26, 2011

Lynne has not improved. She began hallucinating late last week and crying and tearing at her hair. The Docs had to give her two injections of *Haldol* (a powerful anti-psychotic drug) to calm her down. She is now on *Risperdal* (also an anti-psychotic) and is calm.

She seems to know that I am there, but doesn't smile much anymore. While they were trying to determine the cause of Lynne's behaviour, they ran a series of blood and urine tests. They suspected a urinary tract infection, but there wasn't one. But the ketone levels in Lynne's urine are high. This means that Lynne is essentially starving, and her body is consuming body fat.

Mary Sue, Lynne is my height and can't weigh more than 100 pounds. She doesn't have any fat.

Yesterday when I went to visit, Lynne was in her wheel chair. She was too weak and drugged to walk, and barely ate. Today, she was able to walk and eat, but fought me every step of the way. It took me an hour to get 1/2 a glass of her food supplement into her.

I think that on some level Lynne has decided that she has had enough, and it is time for her to go. I remembered what Deborah had told me a while back. She said, "Tom, someday you are going to have to give her permission to leave, so that when she passes on she won't feel bad about leaving you!" So Lynne and I had a little talk.

I said, "Honey, I know that you're tired, and if you need to go, it's OK. I'll be alright, and you can go and be with God in heaven. You can be my angel and watch over me, and visit me now and then in my dreams. And I'll love you forever, no matter what. Don't you worry about that!" Lynne sat very still through all this. Then she smiled and drifted off to sleep. I gave her a hug and a kiss and left.

I came home and told Deborah what I had done. She had done the same thing for her father before he passed on. She hugged me while I wept. Now Deborah is out for a work-out and some last minute stuff for our dinner party tonight. And I'm having a glass of wine while I write you. And more tears. And a nap. Grieving is hard work.

Apr 2, 2011

Lynne has very little personality left, and sleeps a lot. So our visits tend to be short; I feed her whatever I can get her to eat; I walk or wheel (if she can't walk) her back to her room, and she falls asleep.

It has been a little hard for me to find much JOY this week. Lynne's decline has left me very sad. Every time a decline happens, I think to myself *I knew it was coming; next time I'll be ready, and it won't be so hard.* But that's just me lying to myself. It always makes me very sad.

Sun, Apr 3, 2011

Have you ever watched the movie, *P.S. I Love You?* It's a bit of a chick flick, with Hillary Swank as a grieving widow who keeps getting letters that her departed husband wrote to help her get through life, before he passed on. It is very charming, and apparently much too close to home for me.

You see, when Lynne was first diagnosed with Alzheimer's, she set about organizing me so that I could get through some of life's events. She made a list of friends and family birthdays and anniversaries. She wrote out the menu for Christmas dinner, along with cooking instructions. As well as Dave's favourites for Christmas Eve, and menus for New Year's Eve, Easter and Dave's birthday. Check lists for things we needed when we travelled. Wills. Health Care Directives. She got me organized, because she knew that she wouldn't be able to look after me anymore.

For some reason I needed to watch that damn movie! So I sat with Deborah and watched the first part of it before we went to see Jackson Brown, and the end of it when we returned home after the concert.

Seeing the beginning of the movie put me in a melancholy mood, and Deborah, sensing this, began to ask me questions about my grief, on the way to the concert. She spoke about how hard it had been for her when her father died.

I said, "You know, Deborah, I hate that damned disease! How can you hate a thing? It makes no sense! But Alzheimer's has taken Lynne away from me over and over and over again. First I lost my wife; my lover. Then I lost my confidant. Then my friend. Most recently, I've lost a sweet childlike woman, almost like a grand-daughter, that I loved so much! And someday soon, I'll probably lose that simple being that remains, and you know what?? I already love her too!"

Deborah suggested a while ago that I write Lynne's obituary and a eulogy for the funeral well ahead of time, before I was overcome with grief. Deborah reminded me of that last night, and suggested that if might help me if I did it now.

So I sat in the dark listening to Jackson Brown's wonderful acoustical performance (just him on the acoustic guitar and piano, singing his tunes) and Lynne's obituary came to me, while the odd tear ran down my cheeks.

When we got home, I told Deborah what I'd done, and she suggested that I write it down while it was still fresh in my mind. So that is what I did. Then Deborah and I watched the rest of that tear-jerker movie while I drank quite a bit of wine...I awoke this morning hung-over, but relieved. It was comforting for me to remember Lynne and to picture her in heaven.

Apr 8, 2011

They just started trying another anti-psychotic drug on Lynne, as she still isn't sleeping well. The dark rings around her eyes seem to be fading, so maybe it is working. I visited Lynne at noon yesterday, and she was sitting in her room, calling out a little, and tugging at her pant leg. But as soon as she saw me, her eyes lit up and she stopped calling out, and smiled a little! I swear she knew me!

I gave her some hugs and kisses, and she lapped it up. When I asked her if she wanted to go for lunch she said, "Sure!" I walked her to the dining room and fed her most of her lunch, before I asked Paula to help out, because I had a 1:00 p.m. meeting. One of the reasons I knew that she recognized me was that she began calling out again when I told her I needed to leave. She wanted me to stay. It was a wonderful gift!

Today at lunch, Lynne wasn't as good. She was sleeping in her wheelchair when I arrived, but she did come around when I talked to her, and she seemed to understand part of what I said. I fed her and stayed with her and held her hand until she went back to sleep. Then a hug before leaving.

Apr 10, 2011

Lynne was calling out and crying when I arrived today, but had apparently had a good morning sleeping in her wheelchair. I stroked her cheek and cuddled her and talked softly to her and she calmed down after about fifteen minutes. I fed her lunch and took her for a look out the window before sitting in her room and just holding her hand and talking to her for a while. She seemed to enjoy it.

I know that she understands a bit of what I say to her, but I think that the sound and tone of my voice, and touch are very important now. I can sometimes make her smile by laughing at something. It seems to make her happy. That's very important to me.

Apr 15, 2011

It's been a pretty good week, all in all. Lynne was a sweetheart most days when I visited. She is in her wheelchair most of the time now, but she greets me with a smile and a little, "Oh!" just like the old days. Our visits are shorter because she tends to fall asleep right after her meal.

Today was an exception. She was calling out and a little distressed, although I did get a few smiles and some laughter from her! So I stayed until she drifted off to sleep; about 1 1/2 hours. It's hard to listen to her when she is upset, but my presence seemed to be helping her, and it's not about me. If I can lessen the pain for her, that is what I will do.

Monday is biopsy day. I've got my fingers crossed.

Apr 18, 2011

I worked out this morning and then visited Lynne. They had her parked in her wheelchair by the nursing station, and was she ever happy to see me! She gave me a great big smile! But she is not doing well. Apparently, she tears at her hair and cries a lot in the mornings.

The staff had her at the front because she does better when she is with someone. Lynne and I had a nice visit and then I had a meeting with the nurse-practitioner. She told me that they had tried all of the more benign anti-hallucinogenic drugs, and that the only option left was Haldol.

Haldol has some nasty side-effects. It can cause heart-attacks and strokes. "So what should we do?" she asked. It is nice to be consulted, Mary Sue, but it is a terrible responsibility. I told Preta that I had devoted my life to my family's happiness. I said that Lynne has had Alzheimer's disease for more than 12 years, and very few people (actually it is less than two percent, based on my research) survive beyond fourteen years. So this is all about quality of life.

Keep my girl happy. Don't over-dose her, but don't let her suffer. So we will try a low dose of *Haldol*, and the staff will try to keep Lynne company as best that they can, and

I'll visit more and maybe hire someone to help out when they are short staffed.

This afternoon, I had my biopsy. *Verrrry unpleasant!* Deborah took the afternoon off so she could drive me home, which was just as well! I was pretty shaky. I joked a little with the surgeon. "What, no soft music and wine?" I asked. Anyway, I'll get the results in two or three weeks. Fingers crossed!

Apr 19, 2011

When I arrived at Lion's today to visit Lynne, I ran into an old friend, Cheryl. Lynne had gum disease and needed her teeth cleaned frequently, and Cheryl was the dental hygienist that Lynne visited. Lynne had been going to Cheryl for years when she was diagnosed with Alzheimer's disease, and the two of them were quite close.

I got to know Cheryl after Lynne was diagnosed, when I helped Lynne get to her appointment. Lynne and I travelled a fair bit during the early stages of the disease, and so did Cheryl and her husband. So the three of us would compare notes on our trips, and update each other on the progress of our children.

As Lynne got worse, cleaning her teeth became a two person job, with me comforting Lynne and holding her head while Cheryl worked. I routinely booked Wednesdays off so I could spend time with Lynne and take her to her appointments. I didn't learn until much later that Wednesday was Cheryl's regular day off, and that she was making a special trip to work, to look after Lynne. I discovered today that she had waited until Lynne could no longer come in, before she retired.

Today, Cheryl was touring Lion's to decide whether it would be suitable for her mother, when she came across Lynne at the nursing station. She was talking to Judy (the social worker) downstairs when I arrived, and Judy flagged me over.

Judy told me that Cheryl had encountered Lynne, and when Cheryl and I began to talk about Lynne, she burst into tears. I gave her a hug, and thanked her for all she had done for Lynne, and went upstairs. She is truly a wonderful woman.

Lynne was having a tough day today, crying and pulling her hair. They are still adjusting the dose on the Haldol and she is distressed. I stayed with her for ninety minutes, and was able to calm her down a little, but not much. It's very hard to see. Even the staff had tears in their eyes. So did I, but I still got a couple of smiles and a laugh from Lynne, between the moans and crying! And that is something.

So it was a tough day for Cheryl and I. Red wine and maybe an Irish whiskey tonight. I'll drink a toast to Lynne. And to Cheryl.

Apr 21, 2011

Yesterday when I visited Lynne at dinner time she was all smiles! She laughed and cooed and was so happy to see me! No tears, no problems... I left feeling elated after she drifted off to sleep. It couldn't get any better, right? Well, it did. Tonight, there were more smiles, but with two special gifts.

When I asked Lynne if she would like me to wipe her face with a warm cloth after dinner, she said, "Uh huh." Then she puckered up while I was doing it, and said, "Nice!"

After that, while I sat with her, she took my hand in hers, and pressed it to her face. Then she leaned over and put her forehead against mine, and said, "Thank-you." Mary Sue, it may seem odd, but I was so happy I almost wept. Two special gifts to remember.

Apr 27, 2011

Well, Deborah and I were "living the dream" over the Easter long weekend. We left for San Antonio late in the day on Friday, which was good because I was able to visit with Lynne at lunch, and she was doing well. Just a Sweetheart!

We arrived on San Antonio around midnight and stayed at an airport Marriott Suites. Had a leisurely breakfast and worked out in the gym in the a.m., and then rented a car (upgraded to a Mercedes; bit of a splurge!) and headed to Austin for our concert.

The concert was great. James Taylor is well into his sixties, but his voice is clear and he is an excellent musician. We stayed in another Marriott Suites in Austin and then headed back to San Antonio on Easter Sunday. Dropped our bags at the Marriott on the Riverwalk and then dropped the car and walked 10 minutes back to check in.

Great place! You could buy wine or champagne from the "take-out" fridge by the desk and sit out on the patio on the Riverwalk and enjoy a drink before walking to a restaurant for dinner! We had a river cruise, toured the Alamo and "La Vallitta" (shops featuring local artists and artisans), had some great meals, and then headed back early Tuesday a.m., so that I could visit Lynne Tuesday at dinner-time. Lots of fun.

Mary Sue, while we were away Lynne came to me in a dream. I know that this sounds strange, but it seemed so real. It was the old Lynne; the girl that I married.

I dreamt that we were sitting and talking, and that I was joking with her the way I used to. Her eyes sparkled and she lifted her head and laughed, and she lit up my world. Just the way she always did. I didn't feel sad at all when I awoke. I felt blessed by the memory. And comforted.

I have been to see Lynne twice since we got back, and I believe that the meds (*Haldol*) are finally working. Lynne is doing better. She is happy, eating well and truly enjoys the Lion's staff she interacts with.

And she lights up when she sees me! She chatters at me and (believe it or not) we have some good laughs together! I think that in her own way, Lynne still loves me. I know with a certainty that I love her. I hope that we have many more days like this before she leaves me.

Apr 30, 2011

When I arrived to give Lynne her dinner last night, she saw me in the hall and began to laugh and clap her hands together! The staff was all smiles. They treated us as though we were William and Kate! They actually took Ruth (Lynne's table partner) away to her room to have dessert so Lynne and I could have some quiet time!

May 1, 2011

Lynne was tired today, but still happy; she just kept nodding off. The charge nurse spoke to me today about getting Lynne some hip protectors. I'd never heard of such a thing, but apparently they are specially padded underpants that you wear to protect your hips if you fall.

Lynne, after five years of never getting up out of her chair or bed on her own, has developed an inclination to get up and walk around! She is quite wobbly and so thin that she has no padding on her hips, and they are afraid that if she gets up when no one is watching she could fall and break a hip. The change in her is astounding! I am so pleased!

May 5, 2011

Lynne isn't doing as well as she was. She is calling out a lot and quite distressed at times. Although it is not as bad as before she started taking *Haldol*. She seems afraid sometimes. It is heartbreaking to me to see her like that.

But there are some bright spots. Last night when I sat with her, she was crying, when all of a sudden a glimmer of recognition crossed her face. She looked at me and smiled, and said, "Li... Li... Like!" Then she reached over and grabbed my sleeve, and placed my hand against her cheek. It was very touching. I gave her a big hug while I choked back some tears.

Today I visited Lynne at lunch. I couldn't stay as long as I would have liked, because I had a meeting in the afternoon. But it gave me an opportunity to talk to the charge nurse. They plan to increase the *Haldol* dose, which might help. We'll see.

May 9, 2011

Believe it or not, after visiting Lynne and seeing her so distressed, a few things happened that gladdened my heart.... Deborah and I went to an Elton John concert on Saturday night. We had planned to leave early, to attend a going away party for our friends Val and Lindsay, later in the evening.

Just as well! The music was *waaay* to loud for an old guy like me! As we left MTS Center, we passed by a young guy standing outside, listening raptly to the music. I was surprised. Elton John is really way before this kid's time! I asked him if he was a fan, and he said yes, he wished he could afford to see him.

I said, "Well, we're going to a party, so take my ticket and have a look!" Mary Sue, you should have seen the look on his face! Wonderful! He said, "Man, my girlfriend is going to be so pissed when she comes to meet me and finds out I've been in there!"

Deborah said, "Here's another ticket! Text her and tell her to get down here so you don't miss too much of the show! And let your parents know where you are!" So that is how two young kids got $300 Elton John tickets. Deborah and I smiled all the way to the party!

Today when I visited Lynne she was much the same. I spoke to the Charge Nurse, and she will be talking to the doctor when he visits today. I honestly believe that she is almost as upset to see Lynne suffer as I am, so I know that she will be a strong advocate for Lynne. I did say that if the Doc had a disagreement regarding Lynne's care that I expected to be consulted before any changes were made. He has a legal obligation to do that.

Tomorrow is Lynne's birthday. It is hard to believe that she will be sixty-three, and that she has had Alzheimer's disease for over twelve years. My son David was eighteen when she was diagnosed and twenty when I had by-pass surgery. I forget how hard that must have been for him.

I bought her a card and I'll take her some roses. No chocolates this year. She can't eat them anymore. The card reads, "To the woman I'd marry all over again." And I would, Mary Sue, I wouldn't exchange a minute of the life I've had with her for anything else. Tomorrow will bring a small smile and some tears, I'm afraid.

May 11, 2011

Deborah heard it in my voice, and read it in my eyes when I got home today. Lynne has taken a turn for the worse. She is at one time afraid and angry and crying. I held her and pressed my faced to her forehead, and rubbed her back, but I could only break through for a few moments, and then she would begin to cry and tear at herself and wail.

No one should have to live like that, Mary Sue. Just imagining the pain she must feel breaks my heart. I found myself asking God to either make her better, or please, take her now. I spoke to the nurse and the doctor has been called. He will review her chart on Monday, and I am going to be very firm about the course of treatment.

Keep her comfortable. She is better drugged than like this. If someone had terminal cancer, they would administer pain killers routinely as part of palliative care. This should be no different.

May 13, 2011

Lynne is calmer now. They started her on morphine every four hours, in addition to the *Haldol*, and she doesn't cry out as much. She still isn't sleeping through the night more than once every three to four days, so she is quite dozy when I visit. Sometimes she looks at me and gives me a smile, sometimes not. I'll take what I can get!

She is having trouble holding her head up, so feeding her is a challenge. The drooping head is a late stage progression of the disease. I don't think it is painful, but seeing her that way in her wheelchair is heart-breaking.

When I visited her on her birthday, I was looking at some old photographs on her wall. There was one of her and me and my sister taken in our sunroom after my by-pass surgery. Lynne looked so pretty and happy. It brought tears to my eyes when I looked over and saw her in her wheelchair. Life has been so cruel to her, Mary Sue! It's just not fair.

Well, at least she has good care, and me coming every day to visit and tell her that I love her—she didn't understand at all when I gave her the birthday card and flowers this year. I guess I'm doing it more for myself than her at this point. No, that's not true! I'm doing it out of RESPECT and LOVE for her! I'm not going to let go of that!

My biopsy results are in and I have an appointment to discuss them with the cancer doc next Tuesday. No hints on the outcome. I don't mind waiting. It is what it is. Deborah will go with me, and ask lots of questions. I told her she didn't need to take time off work to go with me, and I got *the look*! You women must all practise that one! It says, "Don't even go there, you dummy!" It made me smile.

May 18, 2011

The biopsy results were not as good as I had hoped, but not bad either... The cancer is growing, but very slowly. No change in the treatment regimen is needed right now because the risk of the cancer spreading beyond the prostate is very low. With luck, that may be the case for several years.

May 21, 2011

Lynne is more settled now, but she has changed. For a while, she had maybe four sounds that she made, and to me at least, each had a meaning. One was a happy, a kind of "Look at me!" trill. Another was angry. Another was inquisitive; "What do you mean? Huh?" And the best of all was a little "I love you!" chatter that she would make when she first saw me on a visit.

She doesn't make those sounds anymore. She only makes two sounds now, Mary Sue. One is pain and the other is somewhere between being upset and anger. I don't think that she has enough strength anymore for anger.

Judy (the social worker at Lions) stopped me in the hall two days ago and asked me how I was doing. She then proceeded to tell me about an elderly gentleman who used to visit his wife each day, who finally had to give himself "permission" to gradually reduce his visits to every other day, and then twice a week. Seeing his wife in the state that Lynne is in now was just too hard on him.

I'm not there yet, Mary Sue. And I don't think that I ever will be. I doubt that Lynne knows me anymore, but she knows my touch. Yesterday, I cupped her cheek in my hand, and she fell asleep with her face pressed against my palm.

Today, she was in pain. I put my hand against her cheek, and she stopped moaning and looked into my eyes. I could see pain in her eyes, but also some sort of unspoken thank-you, as she drifted off to sleep. I had to wipe the tears from my own eyes, before I left Lynne's room. Its hard work, but I won't let my girl down.

My one wish is that I will have her hand in mine when she passes on. I don't want her to be alone when God takes her. And I hope that God doesn't let her suffer much more.

May 22, 2011

Lynne cannot communicate, so it is impossible to know with a certainty what is troubling her. And her healthcare directive, which she prepared when she was still cognitive, prohibits any intrusive diagnostic measures. Even if it didn't, I wouldn't allow them at this stage. That would be inhumane. So her treatment is very much as process of trying different treatments until we land on one that keeps her comfortable.

I think that she was hallucinating, but that could have been due to either Alzheimer's or pain or both. The *Haldol* helped, but not as much as the morphine. *Haldol* is an antipsychotic drug. *Morphine* is for pain. They will increase the morphine dose if necessary, but it results in her being very drowsy, and then she doesn't eat much. It is a difficult balance, but her comfort needs to be paramount.

Some happy news...

This is Deborah's "birthday weekend." She will be fifty-seven while I'm away, so we're celebrating early. I got her a dozen roses and a gift certificate to Ten Spa (pedicure, manicure, champagne and dessert) and left them on the table for her on Friday, along with a note "writing off" her share of the condo renovation costs (about $8k) as a contribution to the Deborah Palmer Retirement Fund!

She got a kick out of that! I took her to Tre Visi (high end Italian) Friday night, and to Segovia (Spanish influence, very good) for tapas (she loves to sit at the bar and watch Adam cook) on Saturday night. Tonight I'll cook her a nice dinner. I'm pretty good in the kitchen!

It's a rainy weekend here, and the air smells wonderful. After I visit Lynne, I'm going to finish up some extra wiring in the crawlspace. I bought a forty inch flat screen for Deborah's "den" at Christmas, and I've been a little tardy installing it on the wall! Fortunately, she is a patient woman...

Author's Note: At this point I left for Indian Wells for a few days to check out the condo renovations and do some finishing touches; I almost missed my plane home.

May 31, 2011

I had a safe trip home, with a few anxious moments. Time sort of got away on me on Monday morning, and I almost missed my plane! I dropped the rental car (roared into the Dollar line and threw the keys at the check-in guy) at about twelve-thirty p.m....) and RAN for the United check-in!!

The plane was scheduled to leave at one p.m., and by the time I checked in they weren't issuing boarding passes. So I gave the lady at the desk my nicest smile and begged for mercy! She asked if I had luggage to check, to which I answered, "No!" and then she gave me my boarding passes and called the gate and said, "We've got a runner!"

I cleared security and got to the gate just as boarding was concluded. All this excitement entitled me to a couple of Fat Tire beers with my salad at Wolfgang Puck's in Denver! So I almost had an extra day in Palm Springs! Not what I needed when I had a day full of meetings scheduled today! The rest of the trip was uneventful.

Deborah (bless her soul) said that she wasn't angry that I had almost missed the plane, but said that she would have been very disappointed if I hadn't made it home yesterday. I guess she missed having me around. That was nice to hear.

When I used to travel a lot on business, Lynne would get pretty upset when I didn't make it home when I was supposed to. Sometimes it would be business that would delay a return, or weather or overbooking.

To be fair to Lynne, back when I was consulting, and later when I served on Boards, it happened a lot, and I guess the combination of missing me and looking after Dave on her own was tough for Lynne. She was a wonderful wife, and the only regret that I have about our relationship is that I think I could have been a better husband now and then...

When I visited Lynne tonight, she was doing a little better than when I left, and I got a couple of smiles from her after dinner before she nodded off. I don't think that she knew me, but the fact that I made her happy is all that matters.

The *morphine* must be working. She seems more settled that before, and is eating better. But if I have learned anything, it is that her condition is very changeable. I can't let myself hope that she is out of the woods for now. It is too painful when she takes a turn for the worse. I'll just enjoy the good days when they come along...

June 1, 2011

Lynne was sound asleep when I visited today. I stayed for a while and stroked her head, and then got home a little earlier than usual.

Jun 3, 2011

I received a call from the nurse-practitioner at Lions (Preta) yesterday morning, asking if I could meet with her as soon as possible. I had meetings booked all day, so I told her I would meet her just before lunch. When I arrived, Heather (the Nursing Director) was just getting onto the elevator.

She turned around and followed me to the desk on the floor where Lynne lives. I told her that I was there to see Preta, and she paged her for me. She asked me if Preta had told me the purpose of the meeting, to which I responded, "No."

She then said that Lynne's quality of life had declined significantly since Christmas, and it was time for some hard decisions. Preta then arrived, and Heather said, "I think that I'll sit in on your meeting with Tom."

Preta said that at the *morphine* dose being applied, Lynne still seemed to have some pain now and then, but was generally comfortable. But she was sleeping most of the time, and not eating. It was also difficult to get her to take her meds when she was so drowsy.

So the options were to decrease her morphine so that she was more alert (but in pain) or to install a port in her arm and inject the morphine. If that treatment option was chosen, Lynne would sleep comfortably much of the time until she passed away, likely in a week or two.

Heather said that this had to be my decision, not theirs.

I said that if Lynne could speak for herself, she would say," Let me go!" Heather saw the tears in my eyes, and heard the quaver in my voice. She asked, "But are you ready to let her go?" I replied that this wasn't about me, it was about what was best for Lynne, and that is what we would do—what was best for Lynne.

That is how I have lived my life for over 12 years, since Lynne's diagnosis. When I had a tough choice, I didn't do what was convenient, or what was easy; I did what was best for my girl. Sometimes it was very difficult, but it was the right thing to do, and I could always look myself in the mirror without regrets when I made a choice that way. So Lynne will pass on fairly soon.

And you know what, Mary Sue? The story that you told me about the young boy who almost died, and met his sister in Heaven comforts me. Thank-you so much for telling me that story.

After the meeting, I went to visit Lynne. She was asleep in bed, so I talked to her and stroked her hair for a while, and then left. I held it together until I got back to the car, and then I broke down. Once I was cried out, I called Deborah and left her a message (she is almost impossible to reach by phone during the day).

I drove around listening to a favourite CD until I was composed enough to return to work, to my meetings. Deborah called me and suggested that I go home, but I wanted to keep busy.

After work, I went to see Lynne again. They had installed the port in her arm and she was sleeping peacefully. One of the nurses (Nancy) came in and told me that she had given Lynne *morphine* an hour ago, and that they would keep her comfortable. The staff all know what is happening, and they are all very gracious and compassionate.

Deborah had a client when I got home, so I hung out in my office until she left, and then we had some hugs and tears. Deborah is like you, Mary Sue. She has never met Lynne, but feels that she knows her through me.

Earlier in the week, my buddy Jim and I had made plans to go out for dinner and a couple of beers. I thought of cancelling, and then decided it might be a good thing to go ahead and do it.

I told Jim about Lynne, and he said, "You did the right thing, Tommy!" and then he said, "Ah shit!" and took off his glasses and began to wipe the tears from his eyes. Jim seems tough, but he is a marshmallow. Jim has known Lynne for as long as we've been together, and his father died from Alzheimer's. He gets it.

Deborah and I had a disagreement over telling her family. Her Mom is arriving today and we're having a mini-reunion for her eightieth birthday. Fifteen for dinner tomorrow. I asked Deborah not to tell her family until after the party. I didn't want to cast a pall on the festivities.

Deborah said, "They are family, and you share the good news and the bad with them! They will want to comfort you." I said that this was my decision to make, not hers. We would let them know later, after her Mom's celebration. A couple of days won't matter. She agreed to respect my wishes.

So now we wait, Mary Sue. I'll visit Lynne a couple of times a day, until she leaves me. I've asked staff to call me when her time is near, no matter what time of the day. I would like to be with her when her soul leaves this earth. I want to make sure she isn't afraid, and I want to say good-bye.

With love,
Tom

P.S. Mary Sue—Lynne's ashes are going to be placed at the top of a hill near our condo, and on a beach on the Gulf coast. These are her favourite places in the world. She will be able to see the sunrise in Palm Springs, and the sunset over the gulf. Will you come with Deborah and me in Palm Springs, and say a prayer for Lynne?

Jun 5, 2011

Thank-you for your call yesterday and thank-you for just being you. It means a great deal to me. Deborah chuckled at the thought of you and I and her on the hill with Lynne's ashes. She said, "Lynne's spirit will look around and say, "Who are these two other women? My Tommy's been busy!" But I know what Lynne would really think. She would be at peace, knowing that I am loved and cared for.

I'm sitting in my red chair, having a coffee and the house is still. Deborah is driving our last guest to the airport. We had fourteen for heavy hors d'oeuvres on Friday and a sit down dinner on Saturday to celebrate Deborah's

Mom's (Olga) eightieth birthday. All our guest rooms were full!

Karen flew in from Vancouver. Her husband Rick couldn't make it due to pressures at work, but made up a wonderful DVD of the history of the family including all seven of the children for Olga. Deborah's sister, Lynda, was there in spirit. She passed away about two years ago.

The only sibling that didn't make it was Brad from Sedona. He is self-employed and the economy has been tough on him. There were four grandchildren in attendance, one who brought a girlfriend who seemed to enjoy the party, and told me, "I didn't know that men could have taste like this! Your house is stunning!"

Deborah made a very emotional toast to her Mom. She asked her to look around the room. Then she said, "If you hadn't been born, none of us would be here right now. Thank you for giving us life. Thank you for giving us wonderful lives."

All of the activity helped to take my mind off Lynne. But now my thoughts return to her, just as surely as the sunrise. I'll go to visit her a little later this morning, and this afternoon before Dave comes over for dinner. I wanted to talk to David face to face. This isn't the kind of news that he should receive over the phone. Again, thank you, Mary Sue.

Lynne gets her wings

Jun 7, 2011

I spoke to our son Dave about seeing Lynne before she passed, and he just couldn't do it. Deborah said that I needed to accept that it was just too hard for him to see Lynne the way she was now and I that I shouldn't be disappointed in Dave. As usual, she was right.

I had a premonition that Lynne would be gone soon, so I visited her four times. I went on the way to work, and then met the minister at noon to pray with Lynne. I returned at the end of the day, and then went home for dinner. I changed clothes and asked Deborah to drive me back, as I planned to stay with Lynne until she was gone.

One of the staff had told me that Lynne seemed to be hanging on, waiting for something. I thought I might know what the "something" was. I thought that Lynne was worried about what might become of me after she was gone.

When Deborah dropped me off I said to her, "I think that it's time for you to meet Lynne." Deborah followed me up to Lynne's room. The staff had placed flowers in the room and soft, soothing music was playing. Lynne lay sleeping.

I introduced Deborah to Lynne, and then Deborah placed her face against Lynne's and spoke to her. She told Lynne that she loved me and Dave too. She said that she could never replace Lynne, but that she would do her best to love and care for me, and that she would love Dave, and make sure that he reached his full potential, just as Lynne would have.

She thanked Lynne for making me the person that I am and for raising a wonderful son. She said, "It's OK to go now. I've called a spiritual advisor and they have prayed for a team of guardian angels, ready to help you over to the other side" (Deborah had actually done that for Lynne with my permission).

Deborah left for home, and less than an hour later, at eight-forty p.m. Lynne's spirit left her. It was a very gentle, peaceful passing. I was holding her hand and stroking her forehead when she left.

I thought that I was prepared for Lynne's passing; that I would be able to hold it together. I was wrong. I sat with my faced pressed to Lynne's and the tears flowed like rain. And I thought of all the happy times that this wonderful woman had given me. I sat there like that until one of the staff walked by and saw me. They quickly and efficiently calmed me down and talked to me about what I needed to do next.

I called Deborah once I was able to get it together, and she came back to get me. We walked alone, through empty hallways to our car. It was as though the whole world had left.

I called Dave and asked him to come to the house with Jackie at 10:00 p.m. We had a little trouble locating the funeral director to pick up Lynne's remains, so Deborah called the hospital where she works and got his home number. And we got it looked after.

When Dave and Jackie arrived, we sat and had some drinks, and talked about Lynne until about one-thirty AM, and then they went home.

The next day, I had to talk to other close friends and relatives about Lynne. I had to meet with the funeral director. I had to go back to Lions and take away all of Lynne's things and her furniture. Dave and Jackie helped. I donated everything that I could (including her wheelchair) to charity, kept some keepsakes and disposed of the rest.

These homes give you exactly twenty-four hours to move out. Others are waiting to get in.

The obituary that I had composed was published on June 11, 2011. The photograph was taken in San Francisco about three years after Lynne was diagnosed with Alzheimer's as Lynne soaked up the sights and the sounds of Fisherman's Wharf. The obituary read:

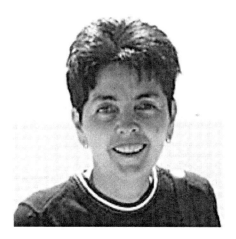

LYNNE PEARSON May 10, 1948 - June 7, 2011
Lynne, loving mother to David and loving wife to Tom, is
finally free from Alzheimer's tyranny, after 12 long years.
During that time, Lynne never despaired or complained.
That was her gift to us, to make the most of the time we had
left. She was very brave. Now Lynne's intelligent brown eyes
sparkle again, and her quick smile and razor sharp wit light
up heaven.

A private ceremony will take place later in June. We ask that
anyone wishing to remember Lynne make a small donation
to one of her favourite charities, the Christmas Cheer Board
or Winnipeg Harvest, in her memory. Lynne always said
that the Christmas Cheer Board nourished children's hearts
and souls, and Winnipeg Harvest filled their tummies. And
as Lynne frequently reminded me, children need to eat year
round. Dave, his wife Jackie, Lynne's brother, Jack and I
miss her dearly. May God bless her and keep her. Thank-
you to all the wonderful people who helped Lynne and I
through her long illness. You truly made a difference in our
lives.

Deborah and I took Lynne's ashes to Indian Wells and scattered them in a favourite location. Mary Sue gave a reading and then we said a prayer and scattered rose petals over the ashes. It was a very emotional moment for me.

I booked a venue for a celebration of Lynne's life. It was held at a restaurant called Terrace Fifty-Five at Assiniboine Park, on June 28. It's the same spot where we had Dave and Jackie's wedding reception, and it had good memories for me.

I invited fifty or so for dinner and some wine. I invited some of the staff from Lions, as well as my Alzheimer's care support group, close friends and family. The folks from Lion's had been key to Lynne's care. I wanted to thank them for all that they had done, and I thought that they would enjoy learning a bit about Lynne and my life before she got sick.

We had quite a diverse group, and not everyone knew one another, so I made introductions, starting with the Lion's staff. I hadn't planned it, but they received an ovation when I introduced them and explained their importance to Lynne and me. It was very nice.

I knew that I was far too emotional to speak about Lynne at the ceremony, so I prepared an electronic presentation of Lynne's life and did a voice-over narrative in advance. The narrative took me a long time because I kept breaking down. But assembling the photos and information for Lynne's story was very healing for me, and I felt myself smiling as each memory unfolded.

I think of Lynne often, and I miss her terribly. But she is in my heart. I was so lucky to have had her in my life. She brought me joy and beauty almost every day. And I know that she is in Heaven, watching over Dave and me.

Epilogue

After Deborah and I returned from Indian Wells and Lynne's celebration of life was over, several folks said that Lynne was likely looking down from heaven and smiling about our get-together. She would far rather have had a celebration than a funeral. I knew that in my heart, so I was smiling inside.

Lynne's brother Jack wasn't able to attend Lynne's celebration because his wife was ill, so I sent him an electronic copy of the tribute I had prepared for Lynne. He was very moved by it, and said that it helped him to recall good memories of Lynne before she became ill.

After I spoke to Jack, I thought a bit about the effect that Lynne has had on my life. Deborah sometimes jokes that she owes Lynne a debt of gratitude for training me so well! There is probably some truth to that—I know that my life with Lynne gave me the ability to love and to appreciate life more fully.

And I believe that I am a better man now than when Lynne first became ill. Alzheimer's taught me some hard lessons, but caring for Lynne also taught me compassion, humility and the ability to love unconditionally.

While I was having these thoughts, Deborah was downstairs working with a client, a young girl of nineteen. She enjoys helping the young ones the most.

During the last week of July, 2011 Lynne came to visit me three times, in different ways. The first was via a check in the mail, early in the week. It was a death benefit cheque from the Canada pension plan, payable to Lynne's estate.

I had to call my bank because by law as executor, I needed to open an estate account in order to cash the cheque. It's a pain in the neck—lots of paperwork! I spoke to the customer relations manager (Jeanette), who had been at the bank a long time, long enough to remember Lynne.

Lynne used to visit the branch regularly when she managed our finances. Jeannette said, "Your account here was set up by Lynne for both of you jointly. I don't think Lynne would mind if you and I skirted the rules a little, if it made things easier for you. Come in and I'll initial the cheque, and you can just put it in your account to offset funeral expenses."

Go figure. Banks never bend the rules, but they did for Lynne.

The second visit was through the life insurance folks, who called to say the "*cheque was in the mail.*" I remembered the talk Lynne and I had about life insurance, years ago. I carried quite a bit of insurance for me so Lynne and Dave would be looked after if I was gone. And not much for Lynne. I told her that I didn't want to profit from her passing.

Lynne's advice was to, "Carry enough for my funeral and a good party, and give the rest to David." Well, we'd had the funeral and we'd had the party, and I resolved the next week I would take my son to lunch and hand him a check for $20,000, from Mom. I had a hunch that Lynne would be smiling down at us when I did it.

The third visit happened while I was picking up in my home office. I still had photos scattered all over the place, from when I put together Lynne's eulogy. And there she was. She was looking into my eyes from an old eight-by-ten taken long before she had Alzheimer's, when we were both young and Dave was a toddler. *Lord, she was beautiful!* I sat there and cried a little, remembering what she was like, and it seemed as though she was looking into my very soul.

That photograph is on the cover of this book...

And ironically, while I gazed at Lynne's photo, Deborah was in her den downstairs, helping that young woman to sort out her problems. I think that Lynne would approve of Deborah.

I see Lynne a lot. Mostly it's good, but not always—a while back, I had a dream (really, a nightmare) where we were at a board dinner and Lynne was not doing well due to Alzheimer's, and she very distressed because she was so confused. And no matter how hard I tried, I couldn't help her. I awoke very upset.

Deborah said that it's just my body processing all the emotions that I've been through in the last while, and that those kinds of dreams will pass. That may have been true, because now it seems as though Lynne comes to me in fleeting moments during the day. I'll hear something on the radio, and it will remind me of a joke or a phrase that Lynne would use, and it makes me smile.

I am remembering her the way she was before she got sick, and how much I loved her. I hope that somehow she knew how much I loved her, when she passed on. It is so important to me.

I completely retired from work at the end of August, 2011. I proposed to Deborah during the summer of 2011 and our wedding date was set for November 12, 2011. The venue would be Terrace Fifty-Five, where my son and his wife were married and where we hosted Lynne's *Celebration of Life*. It was a storybook wedding. We had just over one hundred friends and family in attendance, and a good time was had by all.

I have never seen Deborah look so beautiful. Of course, we honeymooned at our condo in Indian Wells. We visited a bit with Mary Sue, and walked up the hill to visit with Lynne. Lynne has a wonderful view, bathed in sunlight against the mountain. I know that she is not always there. She still enjoys travel. She comes to me often in my dreams and in my thoughts.

I used to have a recurring nightmare where I was out with Lynne in a public place, and we became separated and I couldn't find her. I'd become frantic, because I knew she was afraid and vulnerable. I would wake up very distressed, with my heart pounding.

Anyway, I finally had a different dream. This time Lynne came up behind me in the dream and hugged me. She was OK! I haven't had the nightmare since. I think that she is watching over me, in some way. I hope so. I love her.

Just before Christmas I donated $500 to the Christmas Cheer Board and Winnipeg Harvest (a food bank). Lynne always used to bug me until I did it. They recognize donors in our newspaper and after she became ill, I always asked them to just say, "For Lynne." This year it would be *In Memory of Lynne.*

December, 2011 was my first Christmas in thirty four years without Lynne. I mused aloud that I hadn't thought it would be this difficult for me. Deborah gave me that "dumb-ass" look that women reserve for their husbands and said, "Look at what has happened to you in the last year. You retired. Lynne died. You remarried. You have been through three of the largest stressors people experience in a lifetime. Four years ago, you were living in the same house you had been in for 21 years! I have no idea how you built a house and moved while working and looking after Lynne. You'll get through it. I'll help you."

Then Deborah transformed our home into a very busy place, full of family and love. And that made it OK. I married well. Twice.

Lynne began visiting me again after Christmas. One evening, I couldn't sleep, so I was lying in bed working a few issues out in my head. Suddenly out of the blue, the last picture I took of Lynne at Lion's, before she got really bad, popped into my head. And it made me smile.

She was just a tiny speck of what she used to be, but she had the dearest personality and a wonderful smile! That night and for several nights afterward, Lynne was a feature of my dreams. Most of the time, I couldn't recall the essence of the dream—just that she had been there. She was usually her old self in the dreams, before she got sick. That is how I imagine her in heaven.

Since Lynne's passing, Deborah and I have been in Indian Wells for each of our wedding anniversaries, and we have a little Italian restaurant on El Paseo that we go to celebrate the event. New memories. I go to visit Lynne, sometimes on my own and sometimes with Deborah. Everything is good.

During the spring of 2012, my PSA results started to go up and I decided to be proactive and undertake Brachytherapy. It seems to have arrested the cancer, and I'm happy. I have a lot to live for before Lynne and I are joined again. Deborah will retire in January of 2014, and I am bursting with excitement at the thought of having more time and adventures with her.

In November of this year, Deborah and I went to see the renowned medium, James Van Praagh at the McCallum Theater in Palm Desert. Deborah is very spiritual and we both wondered if Lynne might try to speak to me through the medium. Of course that didn't happen. Lynne was always a very private person, and she would never conduct a personal conversation in a public venue.

But then it did happen. Van Praagh asked the audience if they had any questions. Deborah stared at me with surprise as my hand was raised, as if of its own volition. I had not planned to ask a question. Then a microphone was placed in my hand and the words left my lips, words that had not been formed in my mind.

"Can spirits visit you in your dreams?"
The medium's answer of course, was, "*Yes.*"

Lynne had paid us a visit.

Tom Pearson
Indian Wells
November 28, 2013

Discussion Questions

1. In the **Prologue** to *Please Don't Forget Me*, Tom Pearson writes that *The Alchemist* caused him to reflect on his on parallel experiences. What experiences and challenges did Tom face? Was there a price to be paid? Did Tom (as Paulo Coelho's shepherd did) listen to his heart? What about Lynne?

2. Tom's "Life Legend" in his mind was caring for Lynne. Do you think that Lynne had a Life Legend? Do you have one?

3. Tom writes that Lynne made him a better person than he ever thought he could be. Why do you think that Tom believed that to be the case? Can you think of examples that support that notion?

4. What aspects of Lynne did Tom value the most? What do you think Lynne valued in Tom? What do you value in another person? What do you value in yourself?

5. Tom wrote, "And we lived happily ever after. But remember, 'Happily ever after' takes a lot of work." What do think he was thinking when he wrote these words? Does this sentiment extend to relationships in general?

6. What was Lynne's greatest gift to Tom after she was diagnosed with Alzheimer's disease? What was Tom's greatest gift to Lynne?

7. There are many reasons why early diagnosis of Alzheimer's disease is important, even if there is no cure for the disease, yet. Can you think of some of the reasons? Think about the personal, legal and medical reasons that benefitted Lynne. What actions would you take and how would you spend your time in a similar situation?

8. Tom writes that the Universe conspired to help Lynne and him through various means in the book. Can you think of examples where this happened? What or who is the Universe? Do you have examples in your own life?

9. When do you think that Tom came to believe "unwaveringly in a Higher Power"? Was this a sudden or a gradual transformation?

10. After much pressure from folks in Tom's Caregivers support group, Tom finally has Lynne evaluated and placed on a waiting list for a personal care home. The reoccurring theme is, "You are burning out and placing your health in jeopardy. You won't

do Lynne any good if you are in the hospital or dead." As a caregiver, how do you carve out time in a day to take care of yourself? What support do you need from other people and how can you ask for support?

11. Why do you think that Tom dreams of Lynne? Is Lynne (as Tom believes) "visiting" or is it something else?

12. Tom believes that Lynne "came to visit" at Van Praagh's event at the McCallum theater, over a year after she "got her wings." Why would Lynne do this? Do you think that Lynne was there? Why?

Tom Pearson – *Author Biography*

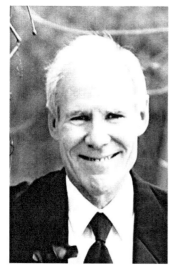

Before retiring a couple of years ago at the age of fifty-nine, I was an executive in the water industry. I hold a degree in mechanical engineering and a master's degree in civil engineering. I have had rewarding career providing safe drinking water to the citizens of Winnipeg, as well as serving on the boards of the American Water Works Association and the Water Research Foundation. I am proud to have been one of the founding directors of Water for People Canada, a charitable organization dedicated to raising funds and constructing safe water supplies in developing countries. Before this book, my writing products were limited to articles in trade journals, conference publications, lectures and a wide array of reports.

But these things in no way define me. They are ancillary to most important undertaking in my life thus far; my role as caregiver to my late wife Lynne. Lynne was diagnosed with early on-set Alzheimer's disease and it was my privilege to care for her from the time that she became ill at age 50 until her passing at age 63 in 2011. This front-line perspective has allowed me to chronicle our lives from inception until Lynne's passing and beyond.

I hope that Lynne's story will inspire you and that in sharing our journey, you find a bit of hope. I can be reached at *tompleasedontforgetme@gmail.com* and would love to hear your commentary on the book.

Resources for People with Alzheimer's

People with Alzheimer's and caregivers need and deserve all the help that we can provide. Here are some expert resources to help in the journey forward. *Don't try to do it alone!* – Tom Pearson

Ten Warning Signs for Alzheimer's Disease

1.   Memory loss that affects day-to-day function
2.   Difficulty performing familiar tasks
3.   Problems with language
4.   Disorientation of time and place
5.   Poor or decreased judgment
6.   Problems with abstract thinking
7.   Misplacing things
8.   Changes in mood and behaviour
9.   Changes in personality
10. Loss of initiative

Source: Alzheimer Society of Canada

Important to Note:
We all experience these symptoms now and then. For more detail to help you distinguish between what is healthy and what are danger signs go to *www.alzheimer.ca* and click on "10 warning signs" or go to *www.alz.org* and click on "Is it Alzheimer's?"

Next Steps:
It is important to see a doctor if you notice any of these symptoms in yourself or someone else. Go to *www.alzheimer.ca* and click on "Preparing for Your Doctor's Visit".

People with dementia can live meaningful and productive lives for many years after an early diagnosis. To learn more, visit *www.earlydiagnosis.ca* and click on "Why Get a Diagnosis?"

If you or someone you know has been diagnosed with Alzheimer's disease or another dementia, it is important to plan now so that the person with dementia can have a voice in their future personal, health, financial and legal decisions. Go to *www.alzheimer.mb.ca* and click on "Planning for the Future".

For more about Alzheimer's disease and other dementias call or visit the website of the Alzheimer Society or Association in your province, state or country. Caring, knowledgeable people at each organization are ready to assist you with information, support and education.

Alzheimer Society of Manitoba	alzheimer.mb.ca
Alzheimer Society of Canada	alzheimer.ca
Alzheimer's Association USA	alz.org

CPSIA information can be obtained at www.ICGtesting.com
Printed in the USA
LVOW08s0100090614

389151LV00001B/1/P